I Want to Age Like That!

Healthy Aging through Midlife and Menopause

Dr. Diana L. Bitner, MD, NCMP

I Want to Age Like That!

Healthy Aging through Midlife and Menopause

Copyright © 2014 by Dr. Diana L. Bitner, MD, NCMP

Cover design by Jacob Kubon

All rights reserved. No part of this book may be reproduced or transmitted in any form or by any means without written permission of the author.

Published by

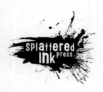

splatteredinkpress.com

ISBN 978-1-939294-27-2

Dedication

To the wise woman in each of us
who is working to discover her
true self and live to her
full potential.

"Whether you are in menopause or just beginning to notice changes in your mood or waistline, this book holds a plan for you.

Whatever your 'that' is, this book will help you define it, plan for it, and show you how to reach it.

Whether your issues include hot flashes, decreased sex drive, night sweats or mood changes, there is 'intelligent aging' and there is 'getting older.'

Aging is inevitable--how you age is up to you."

– Dr. Diana L. Bitner, MD, NCMP

Director, Spectrum Health Medical Group
Midlife and Menopause Health Services

Table of Contents

A Prescription for Infinite Health 1
Chapter One *This is Not My Mother's Menopause* 7
Chapter Two *Surviving Midlife When Good Hormones Go Bad*. 17
Chapter Three *Owning My Own Power: W*A*I*Pointes™* 29
Chapter Four *Creating My Picture of Self (POS)* 47
Chapter Five *Understanding My Place in Process (PIP)* 79
Chapter Six *Feeling Better Using SEEDS™* 101
Chapter Seven *Tracking My Symptoms with the Menopause Transition Scale (MTS)* 117
Chapter Eight *Treating Symptoms with Modern Knowledge*.. 127
Chapter Nine *Creating My Life Action Plan* 143
Chapter Ten *Healthy Aging in an Unhealthy World* 153
Chapter Eleven *A Man's Guide to Understanding Menopause* 169
Final Thoughts from Diana 173
Acknowledgements 177
Works Cited 181
Recommended Reading and Resources 187

A Prescription for Infinite Health

"There is no greater agony
than hearing an untold story inside you."

~Maya Angelou

Are you a member of The Club?

Answer the following questions:
Is my weight becoming more difficult to control?
Am I more fatigued than I think I should be?
Are night sweats disturbing my sleep?
Have I or someone close to me noticed higher levels of irritability?
Have the new stresses in my life created relationship issues?
Am I yelling at my kids more?
Am I experiencing more bouts of depression and/or anxiety?
Has my diet become high in carbohydrates for energy?
Do I have a diminished sex drive?

If you answered yes to any or all of these questions, then welcome to the not-very-exclusive club that drafts new inductees sometime between the ages of 35 and 55. The members of this sisterhood share some or all of the following characteristics: hot flashes, mood swings, loss of libido, low energy, disrupted sleep, dry skin, thinning hair and weight gain. When I tick off the list to my patients, they nod their heads in recognition. "Yes, yes, yes, that's me," they say. Inevitably, the question that follows is, "What should I do?" Do you find yourself asking the same question?

The answer is what made me write this book. There is a lot to do before--and when, the symptoms hit and this book is here to help YOU!

You Are Not Alone!

I am always sad when my patients tell me they feel alone. Instead of confiding in each other about the hot flashes, fatigue and changes happening to their bodies and their lives, too many women minimize the magnitude of what's happening. Often they tell me they're afraid, self-conscious or embarrassed to discuss their symptoms with their kids, spouses, significant others, friends, and more often than I'd like to believe, with their own family doctor.

But the simple truth is they—and you—are not alone. Look around, you are probably standing next to a member of The Club. More than 30 million women in the United States are now going through menopause. Eighty percent of women experience symptoms of menopause for up to 10 years before the end of their natural hormone production and for years after. Many women feel well five years after the menopause transition, but complain they lost ten years of their life. I have even heard women's health specialists say that even though they have taught women's health for years, they are surprised by how difficult menopause is!

I want to engage and inspire women to make better lifestyle changes through proven, evidence-based health strategies, methods I've developed through my practice, and tips to tackle health issues that arise—nutritional deficiencies, weight gain, low energy, sleep problems, etc.

My vision is to see women age healthfully and vibrantly without chronic illness, cancer, or pain, by using their dreams and goals as motivation to make good daily choices.

How women react to their changing bodies is something I feel passionate about as I try to raise these conversations—to confront midlife health before symptoms appear. My goal is to help you and other women discover their best selves by understanding your individual challenges and developing successful methods of dealing with them. It's about making choices that will place you on the path that is best for you, your body and your lifestyle.

Who Am I?

Besides being a physician, surgeon, and women's health care advocate, I am the 48-year-old wife of a successful world-traveling husband, a mother of three teenagers and caretaker of a 100 lb. German Shorthaired dog. My weight fluctuates and sometimes I yell at my kids. But as a fellow traveler through menopause, I am committed to guiding you on this journey and empowering all women—myself included—to make the changes that will improve our health before, during and after menopause.

In my 20 years as an OB/GYN, I've delivered over one thousand babies, diagnosed and treated all manner of gynecological problems, conditions and illnesses. I've performed countless surgeries and dealt with life and death situations. I've worried with my patients, held their hands through difficult times, and been blessed to witness remarkable healing and courage.

I've watched girls transition to womanhood and helped women become mothers. I've also supported my patients through the emotional stresses of marriage, parenting, managing career and home, divorce and loss, while coping with the physical changes that are part of life. Along the way, I became a Certified Menopause Practitioner so I could educate my patients about the physical changes of midlife, and arm them with tools to ensure they choose the healthiest road into the middle years and beyond.

Dr. Diana L. Bitner, MD, NCMP

One thing I have learned from the front lines of women's health care is that: There is "intelligent aging" and "just getting older." I wrote this book to help women prepare themselves physically and mentally for the road into and out of menopause and midlife. As a physician who has spent her life dealing with women's issues, I've always been passionate about translating the medicine and science I know into language my patients can use and understand. I advocate do-it-yourself preventative medicine. By that, I mean adapting your habits and lifestyle so you can travel along the path of wellness into the future.

My goal is to educate, motivate, and inspire women to take charge of their life and health; to review their lives and revive or transform themselves into vibrant, energetic and healthy individuals. I want to give women the knowledge and options they need to redefine their middle years, to reframe their lives and redirect their goals. Each of us, whatever our unique situation, can avoid many unnecessary health problems by being brave enough to acknowledge what lies ahead and courageous enough to make our future health a priority. Making changes now will make "the change" so much easier.

I Want to Age Like That will take the mystery out of how to age well.

In this book you will find information that distinguishes itself from existing books by:

Introducing you to my innovative and unique W*A*I*Pointes™ that provides actionable adaptations and incremental lifestyle changes you can adopt gradually and with confidence.

Giving you tools to formulate a personalized blueprint of achievable ways to manage and mitigate the impact of all phases from pre to peri to post-menopause.

Giving you up-to-date information on how to manage the current health system and how to interact with physicians.

Presenting a plan that inspires you and encourages you to celebrate the phases of life, reenergize your dreams and control your life path.

Changes in a woman's body as she ages are unavoidable, but they are manageable. I'm here to help each of you achieve your best age at any age. Consider me your menopause buddy, guide and confidant.

Welcome to the journey,
Dr. Diana L. Bitner, MD, NCMP

Chapter One

This is Not My Mother's Menopause

> "It is not just that knowledge is power,
> it is the use of that knowledge which brings power."
>
> ~Dr. Vivian Pinn, MD

Patient Tonya K. is dreading menopause. The 48-year-old from Grand Rapids, MI, watched her mother's memory falter and go through mood changes as she went into menopause.

"If my mother even spoke of it at all, she whispered euphemisms in hushed tones: 'I'm going through my change,' she would say. But she was never talking to me. Those were conversations I overheard as she shared with a friend. And, when I got my period, it was not a topic my mother and I would ever discuss. It was part of the mystery my mom revealed only to her closest friends behind closed doors.

"Now, every time I get my period I say to myself, yes! I'm so relieved! I do not have to worry about my memory yet..."

My Mother, Myself?

Tonya isn't alone. Many women recall (with apprehension) their mother's horrific headaches, hot flashes, sleepless nights, erratic mood swings, thinning hair, sagging skin, and wrinkles. Many of us may remember the pads our moms wrapped in Kleenex and stuffed into the waste basket next to the toilet, pretending her feminine life cycle didn't exist. And now, as you approach midlife, the thought of suffering through your mother's personal nightmare may leave you panicked.

Many of our mothers didn't dare speak about "the change," even to their doctors. But that was then, and this is now. Today, information about hot flashes and night sweats flows freely. Still, many of my patients fear their mother's account of menopause will become a self-fulfilling prophecy, that the scary health event that was shrouded in silence will be a predictor of what their own experience will be. Fortunately, it's not all genetic, and it's not a disease. There are many things you can do to make your transition through midlife a normal phase of your life.

The good news is that today women are quite open and well-informed. We don't have to become overwhelmed or define menopause in terms of losses—loss of fertility, sex appeal, vitality and zest for life—as our mothers did. Perceptions like these undermine self-esteem and, still today, keep some women silent and embarrassed to discuss menopause, and unwilling to seek treatment that would alleviate discomfort and a litany of health woes.

As women approaching menopause, we are different than our mothers. There have been major changes in our roles within our families, in the workplace, and in society. We have new attitudes regarding aging. We strive to stay youthful and healthy. We do not want to feel old, look old, or even acknowledge we are getting older. Our lives are much more complicated than our mothers' lives were. There are many demands on our time, from raising children, helping aging parents, working outside the home, and being the best spouse we can be. When our bodies start changing, it really throws us off.

It is my frustration with the out-dated stereotypes that has led me to try to reinvent how women perceive themselves and their mid-life health and wellness conditions. I get frustrated when my patients tell me they have given up and accepted that they will always be fat, tired, slow, or not enjoy exciting and close emotional sex lives. I wish we all could return to the passion and energy we had when we were graduating from high school and were on fire with amazing potential, and strove to be like the graduation speakers who inspired and challenged us to "just do it."

This has led me to ask my patients a couple of crucial questions:

> "What did you dream of when you were 13 or 18 or 22?"
> "How did you start out your life and has it turned out the way you planned?"

These are questions we need to ask ourselves as we travel through midlife. These are questions that differentiate modern menopause from our mother's menopause.

And so I say it again: This is not your mother's menopause! By lifting the veil and revealing the truth about what happens to our bodies in midlife, we can pay attention to the symptoms and take care of them. Before you can break out and get away from the heavy clout of your mother's menopause, you need to understand what is going on in your body.

Periods, Perimenopause and Menopause Explained

Periods or Menstrual Cycles

Let's break it down. Our monthly rhythm is a function of our brains and ovaries talking to each other. Through a series of hormone releases, each depending on the other, the lining of the uterus builds up to get ready for a pregnancy. If there is no pregnancy, there is no feedback for the lining to stay intact and it falls off, hence the menstrual flow. If the hormones are not in balance (poor communication of the organs), either the period can come later, earlier, or not at all. The lining can build up in excess and lead to very heavy flow, shed off in layers and change in amount and color, or not develop well and be very light.

Perimenopause

Perimenopause is defined by a change in menstrual cycles. Usually the first change a woman notices is that the period starts a little earlier and might be a little heavier. The periods might revert to normal and then six months later change again. The next phase is marked by skipping a period or two. It is smart to check for a surprise pregnancy, but it usually just means the egg wasn't great quality that month.

<u>Warning signs to watch for</u>: If the flow becomes heavy to the point of changing a pad per hour, soiling sheets or clothing, or interfering with lifestyle, it is time to be evaluated. These changes can be simply hormonally based and tell you where you are in your process. However, when quality of life is sacrificed, intervention is possible. After blood tests to rule out thyroid dysfunction or altered levels of prolactin (a brain chemical that is put out by hormone's mother gland; if it gets altered, it can cause female issues, such as irregular periods and breasts leaking), an ultrasound should be done to evaluate your pelvic organs, the uterus and ovaries.

Bleeding Danger Signs

- Periods lasting more than seven days
- Periods closer than 14 days apart
- Bleeding necessitating changing products (tampons and/or pads) more than every hour

- No bleeding for three months -- could be menopause or hormone imbalance leading to pre-cancer growth inside the uterus

<u>Treating abnormalities</u>: If abnormalities such as fibroids are seen, these can be dealt with by your physician. However, if all appears normal, treatment would include observation and nutritional support to make up for lost iron in the blood flow and to avoid resultant fatigue, versus hormonal support to even out the cycles. Sometimes a D&C (Dilation and Curettage) is needed to definitively diagnose the cause of bleeding, and to rule out cancer or pre-cancerous changes. Surgical methods such as ablation or hysterectomy could be appropriate, or the use of a progesterone-containing IUD.

About 40% of women have significant symptoms between 39 and 51 years of age. The median age of early perimenopause is 48, and the median age of late perimenopause, marked by missing 60 days without a period, is 49.

Early signs of midlife and perimenopausal changes can start as young as 35, but not everyone knows it can start this early. These early signs include the following:

- Weight gain

- Increased belly fat—also called the "menopot"

- Fat flaps on our backs

- Sagging breasts

- Sleep issues

- Decreased sex drive

- Feeling dizzy

- Feeling tired

- Dry eyes

- Hot flashes

- Night sweats

- Crying jags or depression

- Irregular periods

Perimenopause is often associated with mood swings and increased risk of clinical depression. An estimated 15%-18% of perimenopausal women experience depression or significant mood swings.

Understanding the enemy is the best battle plan. Our bodies can feel like the enemy when we do not understand what is happening. One patient told me, "If only I had known what to expect...it would have saved me so much depression." Lots of little complaints can add up to equal one big problem. We need to remove the mystery and teach the physiology, so the body can once again feel like a trusted friend and part of the solution.

Perimenopausal women are the ones who show up in my office, often driving miles to see me. Unfortunately, too many are already obese, smoke, have unhealthy diets and preventable health issues, such as hypertension and diabetes. They feel their worlds are spinning out of control. And often, they are. The cycle can be vicious, starting with poor sleep and progressing to mood changes, food cravings, and irritating hot flashes. They're looking for a quick fix, a way to "get off the roller coaster."

My goal is to help perimenopausal women tap into their deeper selves. I ask where they are, how healthy they want to be, and then map out a plan for reaching that goal. We talk openly and honestly, and remove the stereotypes that defined our mother's menopause. The goal is to decrease long-term illness, disability and dependency on medication. As it turns out, it isn't that hard. We just need to step back, regain perspective and make a plan.

Menopause

Menopause is the end stage of the change. It means that you have not had a period for more than one year.

During this transition, it's important to watch for depressive symptoms, including anxiety, lack of interest in usual activities, irritability and sometimes uncontrollable irritability. In addition, sleep issues and hot flashes can occur and are often associated with mood changes. Add midlife events such as helping to care for aging parents, raising teenagers, economic uncertainty, job changes and so on, and you can have a recipe for disaster. Mood changes during this transition are real—not imagined—and many, if not most, are very treatable.

Menopause is defined as the final menstrual period and is usually confirmed when a woman has missed her period for 12 consecutive months. So if you missed your period for six months, then get it again, the clock starts over and you are not in menopause. Most women experience menopause around 52.

The perimenopause/menopause transition is the period of time lasting from the first changes in regular menstrual cycles to absence of menses. It's often associated with mood swings and increased risk of clinical depression.

In the Middle Ages, women were burned at the stakes, and even today, some doctors treat this midlife stage as if women are crazy;

they start pushing anti-anxiety pills at them and send them out the door.

The response is understandable. After all, what is appealing about a stage of life punctuated by a long list of discomforts you heard your mom or older friends talking about: night sweats, foggy brain, exhaustion at work, decreased sex drive, bad moods, and hard-to-get-rid-of belly fat?

We do not have to have our Mother's Menopause!

We want you to enjoy this time in your life. It can be a great time in that you have now survived the business of choosing and developing a career, perhaps raising a family, and establishing a household. Now, it is time to ask, "What about me?" If you feel good, midlife can be a great time to re-examine your dreams and make good on the creative promises you made to yourself. For many women, midlife is also the last chance to stop diseases, such as obesity and heart disease, from happening to them. It can also be the last time to make a real difference in how you will look, feel, and be able to function when you are 60 and beyond.

How? By helping you ascertain if you are in a good place and poised for the healthy future you want, or if you're facing a path of chronic medical problems punctuated with numerous doctor visits, prescription medicines, and symptoms of pain, fatigue and anxiety.

A Baker's Dozen of Reasons for Embracing and Celebrating Menopause

Having a healthy body through menopause starts with positive thinking and continues with healthy lifestyle choices. Women often are so focused on the negative changes they perceive, we forget to remember there are many menopausal changes we can feel good about. Here are some positive ways to think about your menopause experience and what lies beyond:

1. Menopause is your new normal.
2. Changes are slow and steady and fairly predictable—if you are prepared.
3. Menstrual cramps are gone.
4. Periods are gone.
5. Menstrual headaches are gone.
6. Cycle mood changes are gone.
7. Increased health insights about menopause make it much more manageable and treatable today than it was for our mothers.
8. Children are most likely grown up or on their way, giving you more time to focus on your own life, personally and professionally. It's finally your turn to ask, "What about me? Am I making a difference with my life? Am I working toward the goals I harbored as a young adult?"
9. Gone are the ups and downs and confusing physical health fluctuations. You're off the roller coaster and experiencing a new steady.
10. It's a fresh start, an opportunity to reinvent you.
11. You are powerful and in charge of your health and your relationships.

12. Sex is pregnancy free and you do not need birth control.

13. Knowledge has equipped you to deal with the challenges of weight gain and vaginal dryness.

Chapter Two

Surviving Midlife When Good Hormones Go Bad

"Each woman is the expert on her own body – and she benefits most if she's well informed. The primary message for a woman at this stage of life is that she can enjoy her body well into old age, provided she makes informed, responsible choices."

~The North American Menopause Society (www.menopause.org)

Hot flashes, night sweats, sleeplessness, anxiety, clamminess, bloating, sudden tears, crashing fatigue, and difficulty concentrating-- it's enough to make a woman go crazy.

"Well let me tell you," Deb, 46, said. "That's exactly how I felt. It was nuts. I thought I was losing my mind. I was so frightened I didn't know what to do or what was going on."

But then it got even worse. She had hot flashes all the time. She couldn't sleep and the early morning anxiety attacks left this writer and mom of one in a perpetually uncomfortable and clammy state.

At the same time, there was a lot of stress with her writing business. Longtime clients were being hit by the recession and writing projects started drying up. Her son was entering kindergarten, going off on the bus and away from the influence she had on his life in preschool.

What was most disturbing of all was that her natural optimism had deserted her.

Suddenly she found herself looking at other women her age and thinking, "I'm the only person going through this. I don't see the misery on their faces, like I see on mine every time I look in the mirror. What is their secret?"

Deb is not alone. Like many of the patients I see, many women are woefully unprepared for the change. That makes sense given the negativity surrounding menopause.

"I went to my primary doctor, and he talked to me for about 10 minutes, and prescribed an antianxiety drug," Deb said. "I was like, 'Really? Is that all you are going to do?'"

That led her to see her OB/GYN who was a tad more compassionate. He ran her through a battery of tests, but they all came back negative for "no organic cause of this."

So, she left thinking it was all in her head.

Finally she found her way to our door, upset about her wildly unpredictable physical state. "I was so upset, but the first thing Dr. Bitner did was put her hand on mine and said, 'We'll figure this out and I will stay with you until we do. You are not alone anymore.'"

Like all of my patients, I tried to help her get educated about this time of life, so that she could help herself.

Our goals: Focus on nutrition and get Deb off the unhealthy diet of saturated fats, late-night snacks, Diet Cokes, sugars and caffeine that were triggers for anxiety, adrenalin rushes and hot flashes. We decided she would only drink what was found in nature—lots of water. Exercise also had a significant and positive impact on Deb's mood and inability to sleep without waking up sweaty and panicked.

Going to the gym twice a week, walking daily and making healthy eating choices not only got rid of the anxiety attacks, but also helped her to lose 20 pounds.

The personal goals "gave me more confidence and helped me become a good health model for my son," she said.

Today she feels much better. "I'm not completely free of all my symptoms, but they're better," says Deb. "And I'm so relieved I've begun to feel like me again."

In this chapter, we will get up close and personal with what is real, including why your body keeps you awake all night, why your nerves are frazzled, and why your emotions are unpredictable. Once you understand why your body is changing, you will be able to work through the symptoms to manage the midlife transition. Join me as I explore the science of midlife to help you better understand what's going on in your bodies so you can have a clearer understanding of the information, and you aren't left feeling dazed, confused, uncertain, and overwhelmed.

As a physician and Certified Menopause Practitioner, one thing I know to be true is the mention of menopause is sure to evoke that deer-in-the-headlights response from my patients. I can almost hear their internal conversation, "What? Not me...I am not even close, am I? That's not me; it can't be!" Sound familiar?

Arming yourself with information about the midlife health changes gives you the ability to alter that prognosis and make the changes you want and need to have a healthy, happy future. You can get from point A—"I feel yucky, bloated, tired and crabby about the bodily changes that are happening to me" to point B—"Who's the healthiest, most fit and energetic 55-year-old of them all? Me!"

When it comes to navigating midlife, there are standout winners and unmistakable losers. It's your choice which role you want to take in the journey.

Midlife Health

Midlife and the menopause transition create the perfect health storm. The symptoms that result from hormone changes can make a healthy lifestyle difficult to maintain.

Symptoms of Midlife and Menopause

- Hot flashes/night sweats
- Weight gain
- Lack of energy
- Decreased libido
- Mood changes
- Vaginal dryness/bladder complaints
- Irregular and heavy vaginal bleeding

If night sweats keep you awake half the night, it can be hard to get up and exercise in the morning. The resulting sleepiness and fatigue in mid-afternoon can make it easy to reach for simple carbohydrates such as the fresh cookies your coworker brought in, or the cereal bar you have in your purse. It can be easy to develop a cycle of poor sleep, less exercise, more simple carbohydrates, and central weight gain, all of which can trigger more hot flashes, night sweats and poor sleep. If you are not exercising and maintaining your muscle mass, your metabolism can slow which can lead to more weight gain.

Hormone changes affect your body chemistry. In midlife and perimenopause, the hormone changes can make good cholesterol go down and bad cholesterol go up. Lower estrogen can make you more insulin resistant, which leads to higher insulin levels, sugar cravings, and fat storage in your belly. Your physiology or body chemistry changes, as do your hormones. This time is well known by women's health researchers to be the time when your risk factors really start to increase for diabetes, heart disease, and stroke. Being overweight, especially in your mid-section, is the basis for these diseases.

In perimenopause, hormone levels start to fluctuate. These unstable levels cause changes in your cycle. One month you'll ovulate normally, and your period will come on schedule. The next month you do not ovulate, your hormones are out of balance, your period will come very early or very late, and you could have acne flare-ups or worsening migraines. The one constant during perimenopause is that nothing is consistent or happens as you had grown to expect. Your body changes from month to month and day to day.

The first step to getting treatment is to acknowledge what is happening to your body. Too often women feel something isn't right but they do not know what is happening. They are sensing the changes that signal menopause, but do not have the facts or big picture to put it all together. And too often, fear makes it hard to face the facts. They are in denial about what really is going on.

You Don't Have to Struggle

Too many women are struggling needlessly. I tell my patients and the many audiences I address through presentations and on my radio program, that if you don't have "it" figured out by menopause, everything gets ten times harder. We women have a choice in how we age, and the groundwork must be laid out before our natural hormone production stops.

Perimenopausal symptoms, which are the warning signs and clues that typically drive patients into my office, are the signals to get it together. Some women come to me thinking they need hormone augmentation or replacement. We figure out the best and safest route.

Hot flashes/Night sweats

Hot flashes and night sweats are the most common symptoms of perimenopause. Early in the process, you might think your night sweat was just that you buried yourself under too many blankets, or set the thermostat too high, or your bed partner was too warm. But when the daytime flashes hit, leaving you red-faced and embarrassed in the middle of a workplace meeting, it becomes quite clear what is happening.

Blame it on the hormones. Fluctuating estrogen levels can wreak havoc on your body and send your inner thermostat spiraling out of control.

As women age and move toward menopause, our levels of estrogen, the main female hormone, begin to drop. Estrogen is something of a biological busybody. In addition to its major role in our sexual development and maturation, regulating periods, fertility and pregnancy, it affects many other processes in the body.

Estrogen plays a role in bone health by helping lower cholesterol, keeping our skin supple and regulating our internal thermostat. When estrogen levels decline, our thermostats become more sensitive to changes in body temperature. This increased sensitivity or intolerance is further exacerbated by anxiety, sleep deprivation and stress. When this overheating occurs during the day, we call it a hot flash. When this uncontrollable overheating occurs at night, it's called a night sweat. Hot flashes and night sweats are annoying, uncomfortable and sometimes embarrassing, but they are not medically harmful.

The best way to stay cool when hot flashes and night sweats happen is to be prepared. The symptoms are usually worse before a period, in times of stress, and, initially, worse at night. Other triggers include caffeine, simple sugar, alcohol, a diet high in saturated fat, mild dehydration, as well as a sudden burst of activity.

Five Foolproof Ways to Avoid a Hot Flash

1. Be aware of your triggers.

- Sugar
- Stress
- Alcohol
- Caffeine
- Sleep deprivation
- Burst of Activity

2. Drink lots of water.

3. Look away (or close eyes) and picture three things you are thankful for.

4. Keep the weight off.

5. Dress in layers.

Bedtime Blues

Sleep can be disturbed even before perimenopause. It happens more in women who are already stressed, sleep deprived, dehydrated, not exercising, and not making the time to chill out before bed. When estrogen drops, even a little, it makes the thermostat even more sensitive. I will paraphrase research done by Dr. Robert R. Freedman, a woman's health researcher at Wayne State University: When we fall asleep, we go into deep dream sleep. Our brain is too busy, and the thermostat is turned off. As we start to wake up out of REM, our thermostat is turned back on, and if we are a little too hot because of getting warm under the covers, or our bed partner rolled too close, FLASH! Our internal air conditioning unit turns on and we pull the covers off! Even if it is not so dramatic, we wake up, and wonder why we woke up. Then we notice our bladder is full, or we spend time tossing and turning worrying about the to-do list and not getting back to sleep, and our brain starts to buzz.

Your Mood

Let's face it, being sleep deprived, gaining weight, and having hot flashes is not fun. But more than not fun, the same hormone changes that cause night sweats and sleep disturbance can also cause changes in the brain chemicals that stabilize your moods and keep you thinking clearly. So, it's no surprise that uncontrolled irritability, depression, anxiety, and fuzzy brain often go hand-in-hand with perimenopause. And, if you have had premenstrual syndrome (PMS), or postpartum depression (PPD), you are more at risk for the same symptoms as you get closer to menopause. These mood changes are not your fault and are treatable.

Counseling with a health care provider can help to lay out your responsibilities and stressors clearly and allow you to see with objective eyes. Combining this with the knowledge of your changing cycles and hormones, a plan can be made to help you cope and improve the quality of your life and all of those around you. Perhaps part of the solution is to know when you will be less tolerant of teenager behavior and to count to ten or walk away before responding. Perhaps you adjust your schedule to minimize responsibilities certain times of the month.

Lifestyle factors can be very important and adjusted when needed. You could focus more on sleep than household chores certain days of the month, be extra diligent about your diet and avoid mood-altering alcohol and sugar, and ramp up the exercise. Sometimes the hormone ups and downs need to be suppressed with a birth control pill, or hormones added to supplement when they hit monthly lows. For example, in the second half of the cycle, perimenopause is marked by decreased progesterone. There is also a place for medications which help to elevate your levels of brain chemicals. These medications can be taken all month or just for the second two weeks of the month.

Sex Drive

Not surprising, your sex drive can also be on the wane. Even if you and your partner have a good history of mutual satisfaction and both are satisfied with how often you are intimate, it is common to see the sex mood change with perimenopause. About ten to twelve days after the period starts, our brains release a chemical signal for the ovary to release an egg. This same signal, the LH surge, increases the sex drive to respond to the timing of an egg being available for fertilization and procreation. At the same time, estrogen levels are peaking which help with sexual response. Because of all these factors, women tend to have their monthly peak sex drive with ovulation, midway between periods. The hormones recede, the everyday schedule takes over, and the hormonal sex drive recedes for another month. Men, on the other hand, are ovulating sperm every day and their hormone levels are urging daily procreation.

If your couple connection is strong, you feel respected and desired, and you share a special intimacy, desire can last all month long. However, if the couple connection is stressed by fighting over how to raise the kids, the budget, or who works harder, getting naked and vulnerable is probably not going to happen.

I teach and think about sex drive, or libido, using the analogy of a puzzle. Every person has a libido puzzle, men included. There are about ten pieces to this puzzle, and a certain number must be in place to avoid libido distress.

These puzzle pieces include:

- physical self-image (how comfortable are you being naked and with your sexuality)
- life satisfaction and competence
- hormone balance
- energy
- physical comfort and satisfaction with intercourse (lack of pain, ability to have an orgasm)
- mutual like of each other
- respect and care
- personal perceptions of sex (history growing up and past experiences)
- ability to have time and space for privacy (away from teens yelling, "MOM")

If too many pieces are missing, then sex is not going to happen and libido distress will be high.

Libido distress occurs when there is dissatisfaction about the amount or type of intimacy between partners, or an imbalance in the desire for intimacy. If the frequency is low, but neither partner is bothered, then the level of libido distress is low. If one partner is distressed by the lack or the overabundance of desire, then libido distress is high. If the distress is high and long-lasting, the relationship can suffer or fail. Knowing your libido puzzle can be crucial to your relationship staying healthy and alive.

Dryness, Discharge and Infection

During perimenopause, vaginal dryness; vaginal infection; and pelvic relaxation with the falling of the bladder, uterus and rectum, can lead to incontinence, difficulty in emptying the bladder or rectum. Thus, difficulties with intercourse can create physical challenges. Age, childbirth, hormone levels, overall health, and lifestyle habits can all contribute to these changes. The reasons can be complicated and can be cause for a health professional to sort them out. Once everything is sorted out, a plan can be made. Women do not need to suffer.

Vaginal dryness from low estrogen does not tend to develop until several years after menopause. I mention this because if you have vaginal dryness before this time, then there are likely other causes such as skin conditions, chronic infection, or lack of desire or inadequate foreplay--your vaginal skin can read your subconscious mind. Are you mad at your partner? Instant dryness can be the result. Many women never have symptoms severe enough to seek treatment. If you want to remain sexually active, vaginal dryness can lead to difficulty in arousal, achieving orgasm, or pain with intercourse. Even without sexual activity, vaginal dryness with itching or discomfort can be bothersome. Before trying any over-the-counter creams or potions, it is best to have an exam by a gynecologist or primary care doctor who is knowledgeable about such conditions to rule out common skin conditions such as lichen sclerosis.

Treatment can consist of using over-the-counter daily moisturizers or lubricants for intercourse. Depending on your complaints and situation, your provider may prescribe use of an acid-level balancing gel, steroid ointment for the vulva, local vaginal estrogen which can be given by applying dabs of cream, application of vaginal pills, or a vaginal ring which stays in place for three months at a time. These can be dosed by your provider to not absorb into your system. Again, many women do not experience symptoms which are life threatening or mood altering. But, if you do have symptoms, there is no need to suffer.

Chapter Three

*Owning My Own Power: W*A*I*Pointes*™

"What you do today can improve all your tomorrows."

~Ralph Marston

W*A*I*Pointes™ stands for "Who Am I?" which is another way of asking, "What do I want for my life?" and "What must I do to achieve it?" and "How do I get there?"

W*A*I*Pointes™ combines your aspirations and dreams with your personal statistics and risk factors for depression and disease. It is a focal point and a visualization tool to help you reawaken your hopes and dreams, and reenergize your outlook on life.

The Evolution of W*A*I* Pointes™

My first hot flash happened a few years ago. I was at the hospital and had just bounded up five flights of stairs to see a patient. As I reached the landing, I felt a sudden whoosh of heat rushing up my body from my toes to the top of my head. I was momentarily stunned. What the heck is going on with me, I wondered, as I took my own pulse. That feeling of bewilderment was followed by an "aha" moment. I remember smiling to myself as I realized that here I was, a doctor, a gynecologist, a women's health expert, surprised by a hot flash. If I could be taken aback, I could only imagine what my patients were feeling.

That night, I was in bed ruminating about my first hot flash when suddenly an image floated into my mind. I was standing on a springboard. I saw myself flying toward my future, empowered with knowledge, reconnected with my identity and my core. I saw myself jumping on the springboard, taking off, arms outstretched, feeling excited and ready to embrace the possibilities. My way to move forward was to dive into the opportunities and steer clear of apprehension. I got up out of bed, went into the living room, got a pad of paper and started recording my thoughts. I drew a stick figure woman on a springboard and wrote all the possibilities for the proverbial woman, representing all of the women who were previously held back by the fear of the change, who now did not have to be limited. I stayed up all night envisioning the possibilities and filling notebooks with ideas, lists and visions.

That experience evolved into W*A*I*Pointes™ and now into this book. I realized that if I combined all the life lessons I'd learned as a physician, wife, mother and a woman, I could impact women's health. From that moment, I resolved to create a program for women that focused on midlife wellness. I guess you could say that hot flash lit a fire inside of me.

Next Steps

W*A*I*Pointes™ makes it easier for you to see how every aspect of your life fits together to make you well—or unwell—as you age. W*A*I*Pointes™ principles help you identify your risk factors and outline steps to reduce age-associated discomfort and pain, avoid chronic illness, cancer, and heart disease through lifestyle changes, motivation and medicine.

I believe we need a new vocabulary in regards to menopause. By that I mean a revolutionary way to think about the change, to see it in terms of possibilities and potential. To that end, over my twenty years of experience, I have assembled a doctor's bag full of tools, including my listening ear, intuition, book knowledge, memory of prior patient experiences, surgical skills, and a prescription pad. Now I want to help you assemble your own tool bag so you can problem solve when symptoms occur or you are not feeling your best.

In this chapter, I'll guide you through steps to identify specific health issues related to hormone fluctuations. By combining the latest scientific knowledge with my best clinical judgment, I can help you make choices to alleviate symptoms and stress, and keep you moving forward with energy and enthusiasm.

I'll also help you zero in on the lifestyle habits that seem to be the villains driving us into this vicious cycle:

- We don't get enough sleep and then we're crabby.
- We pump ourselves up on coffee, caffeinated soft drinks, and carbs.
- We don't exercise, because we're too tired to exercise.
- We find the household chores, the bills, and the stuff we're supposed to be doing stacking up, but we're too exhausted and stressed out to tackle them.
- We add depression to our list because it all is wearing us down.
- The hormone changes kick this off, and about a week after our periods, we start feeling better, human again. But then the cycle starts all over again.

The good news is that if we anticipate the cycle, we don't have to get sucked into this downward spiral. When women change this, it is powerful. Though each woman's symptoms are unique, in treating and talking to hundreds of patients who are experiencing midlife health challenges, I have discovered valuable insights and developed a plan to help you make sense of what is normal and identify the health issues that arise. Understanding is empowering. With this knowledge, you'll be able to make choices that improve your sense of well-being today, tomorrow, next week, next month and next year. Together we are going to change your life and help you feel healthier and more awesome.

I made a commitment to my patients and to myself to create a roadmap that we could all follow, a blueprint of strategies to outfox our biology. So, two years ago, I enlisted 100 of my patients to participate in a comprehensive pilot project meant to identify the major health issues of midlife and distill that information into practical advice designed to help women feel and be their best, regardless of age.

As you begin your journey with W*A*I* Pointes™, let this be your mantra: I will not just tolerate my life, I will live my life to its potential.

Areas of Wellness

There is no widely accepted definition of wellness that I could find to use, so I had to start with a list of categories that includes most areas of health that concern physicians.

These areas are the top tier of factors that contribute to your well-being and include most aspects of health and well-being. I am not only talking about your medical well-being, but also how you feel about yourself as a woman, mother, wife, friend, sister and citizen of the world. Each area of W*A*I*Pointes™ is a component of the state of being healthy, created to make the concept of health something manageable you can translate into an action plan.

Once we think about how to define and break up the concept of wellness into nine main components, the next step is an action plan. If our overall goal is to be as healthy as we can and want to be, the first step is to define what we want for our future. What is health care without a goal? It is what we have now—problem-based care, a process of placing band-aids on problems. So, this is new and different—we are starting our health system with you having a plan with a goal defined by you, not the system. The health care provider is a good partner, like a first mate or navigator with maps and tips, but you are the driver, the one who needs to give the car gas, and determine the speed of travel or whether there is travel at all.

W*A*I*Pointes Nine Wellness Categories

A. Ability to be Active

What is your ability to be active? If you want to be active and mobile when you're 60 or 70 and beyond, you have to get moving right now. How active do you WANT to be in the future? Many women slow down over time because of how they feel in the moment, thinking they will move more the next day. They are fatigued, feel out of shape, have aches and pains or are carrying excess weight. Without a clear goal and

> **W*A*I*Pointes Nine Wellness Categories**
>
> Ability to be Active
> Obesity
> Cancer
> Diabetes
> Ease of coping
> Phase of ovarian function
> Good bones
> Heart disease
> Income security

making a conscious decision to work through the hard stuff, it is often much easier to sit down. Many women feel the pain and become discouraged. Do not let this happen to you. Pick one obstacle, barrier, ache or pain, and find a way to solve it. Move on to the next. Don't let aches and pains or self-consciousness stand in your way.

Exercise is one of the best all around preventative strategies and anti-aging remedies.

You've probably heard it before: "A body in motion stays in motion." It's so true. Stick to the couch, and you will likely gain weight and increase your risk of weight-related complications, including diabetes and high blood pressure. And whatever pain you have now will continue and perhaps increase. Assessing your ability to be active allows you to set goals and track your ability to participate in activities now and in the future.

Trust me, if you're a couch potato now and do nothing, you'll spend your future as a slow-moving, cranky spud.

Ask yourself: In the future, do I want to be able to:

- Touch my toes?
- Walk to the mailbox? Walk more than a mile? Walk many miles?
- Lift suitcases and carry groceries?
- Feel strong and lean?
- Recognize fixable barriers such as aches and pains and know how to move past them and recover quickly?
- Hike the hills around San Francisco?
- Ski with my kids?
- Train for a marathon?
- Join a spin class?

More specifically, the category of Activity describes your ability to be active in performing aerobic activity, your strength, and your flexibility. It also includes how active you are in terms of steps per day, as well as number of barriers which keep you from being active.

The Activity category is important for your day-to-day quality of life in terms of what you are able to do. However, it also has an important impact on your risk of heart disease, obesity and diabetes, as well as how well you will feel through menopause. This affects the symptoms of menopause and sexuality.

B. Obesity

Does weight really matter that much? A woman's weight, more specifically her lean body mass, has many implications for every other area of wellness, including mood, sexuality, menopause symptoms, risk for cancer, etc. In the United States, obesity rates have increased dramatically over the last 30 years and obesity is now an epidemic in this country. Obesity is the main cause of diabetes and high blood pressure, and leads to heart attacks and stroke.

We do not all have to be skinny to be healthy and happy, but if you are carrying more weight than you want, it can feel bad and make you feel bad. If nothing fits and you are limited in activity, the weight can make you feel cranky and downright depressed. The problem about weight gain in midlife is that with hormone changes, the weight gets progressively harder to lose. Many women get into a hard-to-break, vicious cycle of weight gain, less activity, muscle stiffness, loss of muscle, slower metabolism, and so on. In addition, weight gain can cause hot flashes, night sweats and sleep disturbance, all factors which can lead to a downward spiral. Obesity may also increase the severity of some menopausal symptoms.

On the medical side, being obese or significantly overweight increases your risk for many diseases such as heart disease, type 2 diabetes, some cancers and stroke. Being obese makes your heart work harder, causes excess pressure on your joints, impairs your breathing and contributes to sleep apnea. Being overweight (having a BMI between 25 and 29.9), can affect your energy levels, curtail your ability to be active, make you stressed and cause stress on your body.

The Obesity category uses four measurements to describe your weight status: weight, BMI, body fat percentage, and waist circumference. These measurements help determine what strategy is best for weight loss (if needed), and help determine your health status and predict your future self.

Your BMI is calculated from your height and weight. For example, if you weigh 150 lbs and you are 5'8", you will have a much healthier BMI than if you are 150 lbs and you are 5'0". The BMI, however, does not help with understanding how your weight is distributed; the waist circumference measurement does that. Central weight gain has implications for risk for heart disease and diabetes, as well as telling us how and why it is hard for you to lose weight.

Your body fat percentage is a measurement of lean body mass. It is not only a good measure of your risk for illness, but also can be a tool of encouragement. If you start on an exercise plan and do not see an overall change in your weight, an improved body fat percentage can keep you from being discouraged.

C. Cancer

Cancer is a combination of genetics and environment. While you cannot control what genes you are given, to some extent you can control many of the environmental and lifestyle factors that increase your cancer risk. These include smoking, body fat percentage and weight, overindulging in alcohol, and eating a diet high in fat and simple carbohydrates. Cancer begins when cells change into angry aggressive cells that do not follow the rules. There are many kinds of cancer, but they all start with the same process. In our bodies, the immune system has policing cells which look for and destroy cancer cells. But if the immune system is not working well, because of overall health or because an inherited gene keeps the police cell from doing its job, the cancer cells grow and spread.

In W*A*I*Pointes™ we focus on the top three cancers—lung, colorectal and breast -- which affect women and the main risk factors for each. There are factors you have control over, and others you cannot change, like a family history or already having been diagnosed with cancer. Even small changes can make a big difference.

Different cancers behave differently. The most common in women is lung cancer, followed by colorectal and breast. There are important factors for you to know to help you reach your goal of staying cancer free.

Risk factors for lung cancer include smoking, having received radiation treatment for breast cancer, family history, prior lung disease, being exposed to radon, and being a female. Risk factors for breast cancer include a family history, ethnicity, history of benign breast disease, high fat diet, reproductive history, dense breasts and exposure to radiation. Risk factors for colorectal cancer include family history of colon cancer or polyps greater than one centimeter in size, obesity, and a diet high in fat and alcohol.

The factors described above are controllable and by doing what you can to minimize these factors, you hopefully can decrease your personal risk for cancer. Have you committed to a future that is cancer free? Do you have the knowledge of what such a commitment means? Has your doctor asked you if you are committed to a cancer-free future? If not, I am asking you now.

As my mother always said, "Your actions are speaking so loudly, I cannot hear your words." So if you are drinking more than 12 alcohol servings per week, your actions tell me you are fine with an increased risk for breast cancer. A second glass of wine at night may seem harmless, but it's not. You must commit to creating a future without cancer and become educated in how you can do that. It starts with the commitment and then you do your best.

In this Cancer category, we use evidence-based medical risk scales to help understand where you are now and to give a clear picture of you in the future. If you do not want cancer and the fear and treatment associated with cancer, then we can paint a picture of what that looks like for someone who is at low risk. While we all know someone who has lived a healthy life yet still has gotten cancer, reducing your risk by modifying risk factors can be worthwhile. A healthy lifestyle now also has power even if you do develop cancer as your recovery could be smoother and your risk of recurrence could be less.

D. Diabetes

High blood sugars and insulin resistance of pre-diabetes and diabetes affect wellness in many ways. These conditions cause many symptoms, such as fatigue, craving of carbohydrates, difficulty losing weight, dark chin hairs, hot flashes and night sweats. They also cause an increased rate of obesity, heart disease, high blood pressure, and stroke. Unfortunately, too many women have type 2 diabetes and many more have pre-diabetes without even knowing. It is happening in young people at an alarming rate, and the average age for onset of diabetes is decreasing.

The good news is that whether you are 16 or 60, diabetes is avoidable in the majority of cases, and is frequently preceded by being obese. It is a vicious cycle. Once pre-diabetes is underway, the process can be very hard to stop or reverse.

I had a patient who was diagnosed with pre-diabetes and carried her weight in her middle. She said, "I do not understand what you are saying about insulin and blood sugar. I just know that I crave bread and chocolate, but I want to lose weight and feel better so I can go on vacation with my sister." She had a hard time making good choices in the moment of hunger or craving, and the very things she craved were causing her problems. So, I changed gears. Instead of talking about insulin and blood sugar, I came up with an analogy for her. She carried quite a bit of weight in her midsection, so I asked her to give me the name of a woman she didn't like.

"Gladys," she said.

"Okay," I said. "Let's call your belly fat Gladys. Gladys doesn't want you to go on vacation with your sister. She wants you to stay home on the couch. Whenever you crave chocolate or bread or mashed potatoes, it is not YOU who wants it, it is Gladys, and her voice is insulin. And when you eat chocolate and bread and mashed potatoes, it goes to Gladys, not to your brain or muscles. And, because Gladys takes all the blood sugar and gets bigger, your blood sugar drops, you feel tired, and think it is time to rest. Gladys is happy, and as she gets bigger and louder and stronger, you get weaker, lose muscle, and don't even want to go on vacation with your sister. So, who is going to win, you or Gladys?"

"I get it," she said. "I need to think about this." She left our visit in obvious thought. One month later, she returned for a recheck appointment. She showed me her log; she had been walking over 5,000 steps per day and had lost 8 lbs.

"Who do you think is winning now?" she asked.

The Diabetes category is defined by your risk factors for developing diabetes and your current level of wellness on the spectrum of risk for developing diabetes. These range from high risk—a diagnosis of diabetes with elevated blood sugar, large waistline measurement, high cholesterol and triglycerides, to low risk—with healthy blood sugar levels, low triglycerides, and a habit of intake of healthy carbs and activity. We can measure each variable of risk for diabetes. Once you have defined how you want to be in the future, we use the same variable to follow your progress over time.

E. Ease of Coping

Resilience is important in survival and has implications for depression, anxiety and quality of life. If a woman is able to cope with life's ups and downs, she can better stay on course to maintain her health and reach her goals for happiness and serving others in her life. Understanding a woman's ability to cope could lead to strategies for stress management, conflict resolution, grieving when appropriate, and improving relationships. By having a short list—or no list—of things to worry about, a woman's focus can be her well-being.

Coping with challenges is a part of life. How well you are able to cope is a vital part of your wellness. Some women cope well with stress and hardship, and some do not. Coping has been studied and it has been shown that women who cope well:

- are able to keep a positive outlook;
- believe they have the right to a good life;
- ask for help when they need it;
- form a community of supportive friends and family when they need it; and,
- do not give up easily.

Studies have shown that people who are resilient are more successful in life and better equipped to cope with disappointment and illness. If you're unable to cope well with conflict or change, then this inability is likely contributing to overeating, bad relationships, and poor performance at work.

Women are under a lot of stress and it's easy to get overwhelmed. Your ability to cope with change impacts how you experience life at any age, including the hormonal changes that accompany menopause. Good coping skills can save your life in many ways.

There are ways to measure your coping skills, first just by asking yourself how you think you act under pressure. We can measure your skills and your outlook by having you complete a COPE score (a validated test to measure your ability to cope), a quality of life measurement scale SF-8 (short form 8 questions), and a PHQ-9 (to assess you for any symptoms of depression). It is also important to understand your daily level of stress. Are you dealing with an addiction, abusive relationship or extreme financial difficulty? As we identify your strengths, we also want to understand what difficulties you have had to face.

If you wish to cope better in the future, and currently do not cope as well as you could, there are things you can do to improve your skills. By understanding where you want to be at a set time in the future, and how you rank now on the coping score, we can identify ways to help you cope.

F. Phase of Ovarian Function

As women age, so do their ovaries. Women are born with ovaries full of immature eggs or follicles. Each month, several follicles get stimulated as surrounding cells make estrogen and progesterone. The estrogen made by the ovary gets the uterus and the rest of the body ready for a pregnancy. Only one follicle out of the bunch will be chosen for ovulation, and the ovary responds with a progesterone surge. Where estrogen stimulates growth of the uterus lining and the breast tissue, progesterone makes the tissue mature rather than just grow thicker. The balance of hormones gets our body ready for pregnancy and makes us feel normal. As we age and the number of follicles decreases, the hormones are often not in the ratios we expect.

Perimenopause and menopause are marked by changes in hormone levels and can explain many of the symptoms women experience between the ages of 35 and 60. These symptoms include hot flashes, vaginal dryness, mood changes and sleep disturbances. Eighty percent of women experience at least some of these symptoms. For some this transition is hard; for some it is easy.

The symptoms can be interfering with your life in ways you do not realize. Vaginal dryness causing decreased sex drive and therefore relationship issues? Night sweats at 1:30 a.m. causing disturbed sleep and therefore difficulty concentrating at work and inability to get assignments done on time? Experiencing mood changes? Is your family wondering where their mom went and who was left in her place?

By tracking the symptoms, a pattern will emerge that you can predict and deal with. It's much easier to help you improve your quality of life if we can tease out which symptoms are bothering you most. Knowing why and what can be done can be the difference between a happy household or one with fights and discord. By educating yourself, making the necessary lifestyle changes, and perhaps considering prescription medications as needed, you can use your knowledge and empowerment as the best treatment for menopause.

One thing is for sure, it's a transition and there is an end point to the fluctuations and constant change. Menopause for many women is a new normal, a new place of calm waters. How long will each phase of menopause last for you? That depends. We can't predict perfectly when your final menstrual period (FMP) will occur, but we can get close. You are likely to hit menopause when your mother did, although your body type and lifestyle choices can alter that timeline. If you smoke, it's sooner. If you're overweight or eat a high fat diet, your FMP may be later. That's partly because estrogen is stored in fat cells; more fat, more estrogen in the system. In addition, chemotherapy can cause premature menopause.

The cycles and changes of Phase of Ovarian Function are important to know, but if you can track your symptoms along with the hormone fluctuations, you will have knowledge and will feel more in control.

G. Good Bones (Osteoporosis)

I like the analogy of our bones compared to brick walls. Calcium makes up the bricks. Vitamin D allows calcium to be absorbed by the gut from food and supplements, allowing the calcium to get to the bones to be used. Some cells in the bones are there to build new bones while other cells are there to break down old bone. Our peak bone mass happens around age 32, so basically the walls are as big and strong as they are ever going to be. The rest of our life the walls get progressively thinner and weaker. So, we want to have them as strong as possible by age 32, and then keep overall bone loss to a minimum.

Osteopenia, or low bone density, may show up at any time and often is seen during perimenopause. Left untreated, it can progress to osteoporosis and is common in post-menopausal women who are often deficient in Vitamin D and calcium. Bone-building cells work best when estrogen is present, and they do not build as much bone when estrogen levels are waning. Strong bones are important to staying pain free and avoiding potentially devastating consequences, such as fractures, falls and the resulting disability. Women who have small fractures in their backbone can have pain that is hard to control and can require surgery and strong narcotics just to cope. Having maximal bone strength before menopause is important to prepare for accelerated loss which will occur.

H. Heart Disease

Heart disease and stroke are the most common causes of death in women. Both are preventable or at least delayed by a healthy lifestyle, smart choices and medication. Many of the risk factors increase rapidly in perimenopause and early menopause. In that way, hot flashes and night sweats can be a gift to tell you it is time to reduce your risks in order to live a longer and better life.

Heart disease risks are different in women than men, and heart disease can be more difficult to diagnose in women than men. Symptoms are different, but the same bad outcomes can happen: heart attack and death. We all need to know the warning signs and symptoms and get expert opinion from women's heart specialists when the answers are not clear. Sometimes special tests are necessary to find heart disease in women. One of the most common symptoms of heart disease in women is nausea. The other common symptom is unexplained fatigue. These symptoms can be so vague, that busy women tend to disregard the symptoms.

The fact that women are more likely to get vague symptoms instead of crushing chest pain is all the more reason to know your risk factors. If you have higher risk, you can be suspicious if a symptom occurs and then not feel stupid going to the emergency room. If you have low risk you might not have to be as concerned.

In W*A*I*Pointes™ we teach and ask about the gender-specific risk factors that might apply to you. It is important to consider your family history, especially whether other women in your family had early heart disease, before 60 years of age, and whether your family has a history of obesity or diabetes. In terms of your history, your current place on the spectrum of risk for heart disease is important. This is determined by knowing some key facts: weight, height, waist circumference, cholesterol levels, blood sugar levels before and after meals, and blood pressure. Other important factors include your current level of activity, eating habits, phase of ovarian function, and presence or absence of depression or anxiety.

I. Income Security

Being secure with your financial plans can have a big impact on your life and allow you to focus on what is important to you, instead of worrying about money. How can you think about a healthy lifestyle if you are up in the night worrying about money? How can you get back to sleep after a night sweat if you are lying there trying to decide which bills to pay? The author of Harry Potter is now richer than the Queen of England and was quoted as saying, "The best thing about money is that I do not have to worry about paying rent or how to pay for groceries—like I used to have to do." In W*A*I*Pointes™, we hope to help you get rid of that worry, if not improve your bottom line with information and resources we can provide.

This Income Security category of wellness is not about saying, "I need more money," or simply talking about how to get more money. This category of wellness is about saying we need to live within our means and have a safety net. It is about taking advantage of our skills and looking at whether we are maximizing our earning potential. It is about taking responsibility, putting fear aside, and dealing with the numbers. It is also about knowing the facts about what your goals are, what your income potential is, and how much money you owe, that can take away your fear. Including financial concerns in a wellness program, is giving us the power to add it to wellness instead of take away. Feeling organized and living within your means feels more secure than buying more stuff than you can afford and then trying to figure out how to pay the credit card bills.

Suze Orman, a well known American financial expert, relates a story about a time early in her career when she was sitting in a diner and looking at the waitress thinking that the waitress (who presumably had a smaller income than Orman), was probably richer than she was and certainly less stressed to not be carrying huge debt. Orman was dealing with debt at the time, and experienced an epiphany that day about the value of being debt free, living within your means, and having a safety net. If you do not have the skills to figure this out on your own, ask for help! Deciding you need help is the first step.

W*A*I*Pointes™ Summary

W*A*I*Pointes™ is about common sense and putting knowledge to work for you. It is about taking all the information out there and organizing it to fit your situation, your health, and your desires for your future. You've now met the W*A*I*Pointes™ Nine Wellness Categories. I'm not here to tell you what to do, but instead to help you decide what you want to do and help you understand that the choices you make today dramatically impact how well you live tomorrow, next week, next month or into the next decade. I can't offer any magical solutions, but I can offer a common sense approach to wellness by going back to the basics.

Chapter Four

Creating My Picture of Self (POS)

"The first step to getting the things you want out of life
is this: Decide what you want."

~Ben Stein

It was a normal day in the office, and I was in my usual rush to keep moving between patient rooms when I almost collided with a woman I didn't recognize. I smiled, apologized for almost knocking her down, and continued to race toward the next room.

"Remember me and what you asked me last year?" she asked. "You asked me how I wanted to be at 50."

I stopped, confused, but now curious.

"It took me awhile to come up with the answer, but I finally figured it out. I decided I wanted to be hot and now I am!"

Standing in front of me was a long-time patient with a brand new fresh look and outlook. This was the new and improved woman in the way she envisioned change for herself. In the twelve months since her last physical exam, she had regrouped, reinvented and was forging ahead with new purpose. At age 50, she gained energy, lost weight and went from a size 12 to a size 6. She was in training for a half-marathon and along the way had figured out what "it" meant for her.

She had visualized the person she wanted to become and the life she wanted to live, and in one year, she had made a major milestone in achieving her goals of wellness, happiness and being who she was meant to be.

Her healthy transformation had started because she visualized herself in the future. She knew that if she continued on the same path of infrequent exercise, eating on the run, and frequent late nights, her future self was not hot. She committed to a new lifestyle all while visualizing her future hot self. Her health success was a gift to herself and her family. Her whole outlook had changed and she was happier because of it!

What is Picture of Self (POS)?

Picture of Self (POS) is like a financial plan for your health. If you were to go to a financial planner to discuss your retirement plans, she would ask you how much money you would like to have when you retire. You would consider the kind of lifestyle you wish for at retirement and figure out how much that would cost. Then, you and the financial planner would decide on a working figure in order to start the planning process. This number is the same as your POS—only your POS is your health goal, how you want to be at a certain age or can picture yourself at a certain event in the future, such as your child's wedding or at your retirement.

Women who approach midlife and menopause with a plan fare best. The plan needs a goal to work toward, just as a map needs a destination. By investing in and thinking about what kind of life and health you want to have in 10, 20, or 30 years, you become a better advocate for your own health and wellness. Patients like the one I bumped into in the hallway know there is more to life than resignation and acceptance. It is never too late to get closer to how you want to be and feel.

Patients who develop a POS for themselves, reengage with their bodies and souls. As their personalized health planner, like a financial planner, I then have something to help them work toward. Yes, I have a wealth of knowledge and life experience to bring to the table but every woman needs her own plan. My conviction is that women need to take charge of their health and wellness as they move through their life in all realms—physical, mental, emotional, and spiritual. The key to staying vibrant and relevant is figuring out how to continually be true to yourself.

The journey can be difficult because midlife typically hits at the same time the kids are leaving home, parents are aging, and self-definition issues are coming to the surface. Suddenly we find ourselves wondering where all the time went and facing the person we have become, and it can be painful! That's why it's important to create and commit to your POS as soon as possible. Can women reinvent themselves in midlife? Absolutely!

You—and Improved

If you have been feeling a little change is needed, you have come to the right place. Change starts with a decision and clear picture of who you want to be at a certain age or at a certain event in the future.

We will start by creating your personal health plan whereby I will ask, "Who do you want to be, as in what is your Picture of Self (POS)?" Then, "Where is your health now and how do you feel?" It will be important to understand your current health habits and perhaps how your family health history contributes to your POS.

The choices—the healthy habits you bring to your life—will place you on a path to deliberate wellness. Between career, family, friends, and juggling life's responsibilities, carving out some precious time for you can be a real challenge for most women.

Having a joyful and fulfilling life experience is about discovering exactly what matters most to you in life and honoring that. It's focusing on achieving your dreams and visions, but doing so on your terms, in ways that fulfill you.

By creating your POS and drawing out what barriers you face based on your genetics and lifelong habits, we can make a realistic plan to reach the goals based on your childhood dreams. Have you considered how you want to live the rest of your life? Have you thought about how you want to live your last days? How do you want to enjoy this challenging world with all of its abundance and potential? There are so many opportunities and yet many people suffer from wasted potential! As a practicing physician, I see it every day.

Create Your Own POS Journal

In Chapter Three, we discussed the W*A*I*Pointes™, which stands for "Who am I," and is another way of asking:

- What do I want for my life?
- What must I do to achieve it?
- How do I get there?

Here, the Nine Areas of Wellness defined by W*A*I*Pointes™ provide a roadmap for creating your POS. Use these categories as a way to visualize and write down the person you want to be and the life you want to be living in a year, or five or ten. Your POS is as important to achieving your goal of wellness as any medical intervention. There are suggestions to get you thinking, but the POS is about what YOU want, not what others want.

Your POS, by definition, is a very personal image and goal. The following questions are meant to get you thinking and guide you to answers which will define your path forward. As you ponder each category, write down your answers in your own words to define your POS.

First, take a deep breath, let all other thoughts leave your mind, and dare to dream forward in time. Settle on a date or event that really resonates with you. Is it the age you saw your mom start to age, or the age your aunt got breast cancer, or your age at retirement when you hope to transition to a time of exciting new change? For me, it is the graduation of my youngest child. He will be done with high school, and have plans for his next steps—inevitably out of the nest. I will be 53, with many years ahead. I cherish my relationship with my kids and feel that if I have my own thing going on and am healthy and happy, I will be in the best place to keep good relationships with my kids. So, I have an overall picture of my POS at that event. If I relax and really work to conjure the image, I can feel what that day will be like—the way my clothes fit and feel, the swing of my hair, my good energy upon waking for the day, the excitement of the day and lack of worry about whether I can afford the party. In describing your POS, I want you to do the same. How do you feel on that day—the event or birthday or last day of work at your present job?

After we have a clear image of our POS, it is time to break it down into categories. Otherwise, it can be somewhat overwhelming when we try to figure out how to make the POS happen. As we go through the categories, I want you to use every experience and memory of family members, TV or book characters, and personal experience to really imagine the possibilities and picture how you are at your chosen future date in each of the nine categories.

For each category there is a description, general questions to answer, and then specific category questions to answer. These questions are meant to get you thinking and to define your POS so you can chart it on your Life Action Plan (described in Chapter Nine).

Dr. Diana L. Bitner, MD, NCMP

POS Wellness Categories

A. Ability to be Active

Picture your goal date. At that time, on that date, what are you able to do? How strong are you? What is your stamina? What is your energy level? What sports can you play? Remember, this is the time to picture what you want. It is important to be somewhat realistic, but it is never too late to have more of what you want, so do not hold back in your dreams. Do you want to be able to hike the Appalachian Trail? Or are you just fine with gardening and being active closer to home? Let's get more specific.

General Questions to ask yourself:

- What is my ability to shop for household items, and for clothes and recreation?
- What is my ability to maintain my household?
- What is my ability to care for my pets and family members, i.e. grandchildren or parents or children—as might be necessary?
- What is my ability to exercise, play sports, travel, stand up and give speeches?
- What is my ability to carry a suitcase, open a jar, get up if I fall down?
- Do I want to be able to swim in a pool, swim in a lake, kayak, or water ski?
- Can I garden with the squatting, digging and carrying of plants that requires?

More specifically for W*A*I*Pointes™, in which category does your POS fit?

3—Very Active Presidential Fitness Score >66 percentile (66%)	• More fit than 66% of women your age • Doing more than 10,000 steps per day or more than 110 minutes of aerobic activity per week • Strength training more than 3x per week • Only the rare barrier keeps you from your plan
2—Moderately Active Presidential Fitness Score >33 percentile (33%)	• More fit than 33% of women your age • Moving between 5,000 and 10,000 steps per day • Strength training 0-2x per week • 1-3 barriers that could derail you from your plan any day
1—Limited Activity Presidential Fitness Score <33 percentile (33%)	• Less fit than 33% of women your age • Moving less than 5,000 steps per day • No strength training event per week • Three or more barriers to activity exist daily which disrupt your chances of activity

B. Obesity

We all get dressed, and when we do, we can feel how our clothes fit and we look in the mirror to see how the clothes hang on our bodies and how we look. Because of this, I believe that many of us think about our weight every day. I also think we all have a favorite weight, and that might correspond to a realistic goal, or not. This is the time to dream and set goals; remember, it is never too late. It can be harder to reach a goal as we age, but it is never too late. As you go through this process, you might decide the goal you chose initially is not achievable by the lifestyle you are willing to live, or the changes you are willing to make.

This concept is best illustrated by a story of a patient of mine. She was diagnosed with breast cancer before menopause, and chemotherapy was successful in treating her cancer, but threw her into menopause and with her hormone changes, sleep deprivation, lifestyle changes as a result of treatment-induced fatigue, including an inability to exercise during treatment, she gained at least 40 pounds. She had always been healthy—thin, very active, and did not have to think much about what she ate or drank. Her weight gain affected her mood, self image, and daily happiness! We spent time talking about what she ate and drank, and at the time of the discussion, she was making healthy choices and had become active again. The problem was that her diet and activity were adequate to maintain the new weight, but not in a ratio to cause her to lose weight. Another issue was that she was not sleeping well, which is known to cause sugar craving and promote belly fat storage—the root of all evil. Based on our discussions, she made further changes, and improved her sleep habits. She lost maybe five pounds, which was not close enough to her POS. Still frustrated, she sought the help of a physician.

Upon her return to my office, I could not wait to hear what she had learned and to find out if she had gotten closer to her goal. She had in fact lost another 15 pounds, which made her happy, but the chief gift of the retreat was to have found peace with a more realistic weight POS. She knew if she totally dedicated herself to intense workouts, a drastically different diet with a period of time with higher protein, lower carbohydrate, and no red wine, she could reach her pre-cancer weight again. However, she decided that reaching that weight was not so important to her. She chose to not give up the glass of red wine she shared with her husband every night, and make food and exercise choices to maintain her current weight.

What is your POS in the area of weight, body fat percentage, and waist circumference?

General questions to ask yourself:

- What is my goal weight?
- What weight can I live with? At what size and weight do I feel best?
- What weight do I feel I can maintain with a lifestyle that fits my current work and family obligations and matches my ability to be active?
- In the future, how do I feel in my body, related to how I carry the weight and how my clothes fit and what clothes I can wear?

More specifically for W*A*I*Pointes™--in which category does your POS fit?

3—Healthy	<ul><li>Waist circumference <35 inches</li><li>BMI <25.0, and</li><li>Body fat percentage in healthy range for your age (20-40: 21-33%, 41-60: 23-35%, and 61-79: 24-36%)</li></ul>

2—Overweight	• Waist circumference 35-39 inches • BMI 25-29.9 • Body fat percentage in overweight range for your age (20-40: 33-39%, 41-60: 35-40%, 61-79: 36-42%)
1—Obese	• Waist circumference 40 inches or higher • BMI >30 • Body fat percentage obese (20-40: >39%, 41-60: >40%, 61-79: >42%)

C. Cancer

What is your picture of yourself in the future related to cancer? None of us want to hear the C word, but have you committed to doing everything you can to not ever have to hear that word? Is your POS cancer free? If your answer is yes, then claim that future!

Too many women just accept the possibility, or worse, the high probability they will get cancer. "My mom and grandmother had cancer, I am just thinking it will happen," instead of, "I am going to learn from them, learn what the risk factors are, and do everything I can to not get cancer." It does not have to happen! But you must start with a POS that is cancer free. Many women do not know about the small changes they could make to reduce their risk for cancer, and some are more obvious than others. Of course, smoking is an obvious risk factor that needs to stop to reduce risk for lung and cervical cancer (as well as heart disease and stroke). However, there are lifestyle connections many women do not know. For example, drinking more than 14 servings of alcohol per week can increase the risk of breast and colon cancer, as well as maintain a higher weight, which increases the risk of breast and colon cancer, diabetes and heart disease. Everything is interrelated!

Before you can start on a journey, you must have a destination. What is your POS for breast cancer, colon cancer, lung cancer, and all the other cancers that rob women and their friends and families of precious time together? Uterine cancer mostly occurs in women who are overweight and postmenopausal. Would you be okay with that? If big enough changes are not possible, at least are you aware and know what to look for? That is what we are talking about.

General questions to ask yourself:

- Does my POS, at the chosen date or event, include fear of cancer?
- Does it include having recently survived cancer?
- Does it include an active diagnosis of cancer and having to cope with treatment side effects?
- Am I, at age _____, feeling strong and confident that I am doing everything possible to prevent and avoid cancer?
- And if I were to ever get cancer, am I healthy enough to fight back?
- Do I ever want to hear that dreaded phrase: "You have breast cancer?" (or lung cancer or colon cancer)?
- What can I do to prevent cancer and stay on track to keep my risk low?

More specifically for W*A*I*Pointes™, we will break down your cancer risk to specifically look at lung, colorectal, and breast cancer. These are the top three cancers of women.

Types/Cancer	Lung	Colorectal	Breast
3—Low Risk	No smoking ever; Former, quit ≥20 yrs ago	≥50 yrs, normal colonoscopy; ≤3 srvgs red meat/week; ≤1 alcohol/day; Vit D & calcium; ≥30 min exercise most days	No 1st degree relative pre-menopause breast cancer; No prior biopsies; ≥30 min exercise/day; ≤1 alcohol/day; BMI ≤30; Screening
2—Moderate Risk	Quit ≤20 yrs, large city 10+ yrs; Long secondhand smoke; Factory wk. ≥10 yrs; Radiation exposure	Hx of colon polyps; Family hx of lg polyps; IBS ≥10 yrs; ≥2 red meat wk; ≥1 alcohol/day; No screening colonoscopy	Family hx 1st degree post-menopause breast cancer; ≤30 min exercise/day; 1-2 alcohol/day; BMI ≥30
1—High Risk	Current smoker; Prior lung cancer; High risk symptoms: changing cough, shortness breath, chest pain, cough up blood	Personal hx colon cancer; 1st degree relative colon cancer; Family cancer syndromes; Symptoms: blood in stool, change in BM, chronic abdominal pain	Family hx 1st degree relative pre-menopause breast cancer; FH male breast cancer; BRCA 1 or 2+; Prior breast cancer; Past high dose radiation; Gale ≥20%

D. Diabetes

What is your POS related to the condition of type 2 diabetes? Do you know what that is and what it means? What do you feel like on the inside related to the happenings of type 2 diabetes or prediabetes type 2? Is your POS smart about the risks for type 2 diabetes and know the signs to watch for? Type 2 diabetes can feel bad by causing sugar cravings, sugar highs and lows, fatigue, rapid weight gain, and depressed mood. It can also cause aging and inflammation on the inside of organs and blood vessels. With diabetes, you are more prone to infection, have a higher risk for heart attacks, feel more tired, crave more sugar, and find it difficult to exercise.

Do people in your family have type 1 diabetes? Are you already diagnosed with pre-diabetes? Did you have gestational diabetes during your pregnancy? Do you carry your weight in the middle section of your body and have a hard time losing weight even if you are following a healthy diet and lifestyle? Have you been frustrated with fatigue and belly fat? What does your POS look like?

Diabetes is preventable. Unfortunately, once you have DM II, you do have an increased risk of heart disease that does not go away. But even then, by getting your sugars under control, you delay heart disease from causing problems and you feel better longer.

General questions to ask yourself:

- What does my POS look like?
- Do I have a little, or a lot, of belly fat I need to lose, or no belly fat?
- Do I have family members with a history of diabetes?
- Do I need to start taking precautions?
- If I had diabetes in pregnancy, do I want to get it back?

- Do I want to live with sugar cravings and sugar addiction? Or do I walk away from sweets, able to have only a taste of frosting or none at all?
- Do I want to feel no control over my weight? Or just see it go up and up and up?
- Do I want slow sugar-related fatigue?
- Do I want to have a heart attack?
- Do I see myself taking diabetes medicines for the rest of my life and maybe insulin shots?

By asking yourself the above questions, you will be able to construct your POS and have a clear picture of what you are working toward, and feel good in the meantime as you get closer to that set date.

More specifically for W*A*I*Pointes™, in which category does your POS fit?

3—Low Risk	<ul><li>No family hx of type 2 diabetes</li><li>Normal fasting blood sugar and glucose tolerance</li><li>Waist circumference <35 inches</li></ul>
2—Moderate Risk	<ul><li>Impaired fasting blood sugar</li><li>Hx of PCOS (polycystic ovarian syndrome)</li><li>Hx of metabolic syndrome</li><li>Hx of gestational diabetes</li><li>Family hx of type 2 diabetes</li><li>Waist circumference >35 inches</li></ul>

	• Symptoms of sugar craving and easy weight gain
1—High Risk	• Hx of type 2 diabetes • Fasting blood sugar >125 mg/dl • HgA1C >6.5% • Random blood sugar > 200 mg/dl

E. Ease of Coping: Resilience

Everyone has ups and downs. The longer I am in health care and medicine, and take care of patients, the more I have learned that everyone has something that is hard. Everyone has a story and has had challenges. But not everyone copes the same way. Not everyone handles challenges with the same level of success. Some women struggle with anxiety and/or depression which makes coping more difficult. For some it is a dysfunctional family, including people who have broken trust and caused harm. For some it is financial difficulty, for some it is coping with children who have made poor decisions, and for others it is health conditions that seem insurmountable. I believe you are more likely to cope successfully with whatever gets thrown in your path if you make a decision to cope well, identify your weaknesses with coping (if any exist), and figure out how to be prepared for the unknown.

What does your POS look like in terms of how you cope with challenges and stress? We all know women in our lives who are calm and think clearly in times of stress. Some women yell, some cry, some hide, some get headaches, some eat or drink in excess to avoid having to face reality, and some face hardship head on. Picture one of the calm women you have seen take on any situation. What does she do? How does she handle it?

General questions to ask yourself:

- How do I see my POS coping with tough times?
- What will happen when my children are older and dealing with their own life situations?
- Can I be a stabilizing force?
- Do I fall apart or get stronger?
- If my parents are sick, how will I still take care of myself and them?
- How well does my future self face life's challenges without letting healthy habits go? What are my coping mechanisms?
- Will I fall into a cycle of not sleeping, stress eating, drinking too much coffee, and yelling at everyone around me?
- At that future date of my POS and beyond, when I encounter an obstacle, can I commit to making a list, weighing the options, keeping a positive attitude, and staying strong?

More specifically for W*A*I*Pointes™, in which category does your POS fit?

3—Resilient – low risk for poor coping	<ul><li>PHQ-9 0-4</li><li>Habit of maintaining a positive outlook</li><li>Honest with self and others</li><li>Established support group</li></ul>
2—Moderate risk for adequate coping	<ul><li>PHQ-9 5-14</li><li>Currently lost positive outlook</li><li>Increased anxiety</li></ul>

	• Some dysfunction in relationships or work because of coping methods • Lost contact with support group, but they exist
1—High risk for poor coping	• PHQ-9 15-27 • Not able to keep positive outlook • Depression or anxiety crippling relationships or work • No support group

F. Phase of Ovarian Function

Menopause happens to us all, whether we want it or not. For some it happens early; for some it happens late. Sometimes it happens gradually, sometimes slowly, and sometimes totally unexpected because of issues like cancer or cancer treatment. The most consistent predictor is knowing when your mom had natural menopause as you are most likely to have menopause when she did. Menopause does not have to be a bad thing, and there are lifestyle habits you can do to make the change easier. For some women, medications are also options, and a Certified Menopause Practitioner from the North American Menopause Society can help you decide (menopause.org).

So, as you think about your POS at the age or event you have pictured, how is she dealing with hormone changes? We cannot choose the timing of menopause, but we can choose how well we cope with the hormone changes which will accompany the ovarian aging process. Part of the POS is having knowledge of where you are in the aging process, and part is understanding which symptoms are related to hormone changes and which are not, and what treatment options are options for you. Is your POS confused or knowledgeable? Is she hot flashing like crazy or is she cool and smiling? Is she the one with the answers at the party, or is she the one asking the questions?

General questions to ask yourself:

- Do I want to experience embarrassing hot flashes?
- Do I want to sleep soundly, or spend the nights tossing and turning?
- Do I want to have to change my sheets due to night sweats?
- Do I want to be even-keeled or cranky? Cry at the drop of a hat?
- Am I moody and irritable?
- Will I cry for no reason?
- Do I want to be able to remember why I went to the grocery store, or forget half of my list?
- Will I have trouble concentrating and finishing what I start because I am so sleep deprived from night sweats?
- Is my POS going to be remembered for generations as short-tempered and 'crazy' as I went through my change?
- Is my POS going to be the example for future generations, using good information and then teaching the women who follow?

There are three main categories of symptoms that occur with the menopause transition, which have been well documented by researchers over many decades. Those categories are: psychological, body complaints, and vasomotor (or hot flashes/night sweats). I came up with an inventory scale called the Menopause Transition Scale (MTS) which is short and easy to use. After years of taking care of women in menopause transition, I believe this sums up the symptoms and covers the three main categories. I want you to consider how your POS is for each of these symptom categories and record your numbers (1, 2 or 3):

Hot flashes/night sweats   _____
Weight   _____
Energy   _____
Libido   _____
Moods   _____
Vaginal dryness   _____
Bleeding   _____

More specifically for W*A*I*Pointes™, in which category does your POS fit?

3—Minimal/predictable functional	• Minimal or rare distress: no or rare hormone related symptoms • MTS >19 • Knowledge of phase and symptoms
2—Moderate distress with some effect on daily life	• Symptoms mild and predictable • MTS 12-18
1—Low quality of life dysfunctional	• Able to sometimes predict symptoms and severe distress • MTS <12 • Minimal knowledge of symptoms triggers, no knowledge of phases

G. Good Bones (Osteoporosis)

Healthy bones support us as we age. Strong bones allow us to keep doing the activities we love like hiking, skiing, horseback riding, and all of the daily activities we take for granted. Strong bones help us live without fear of the consequences of stepping wrong off a curb or slipping on the ice in the winter. Strong bones help us avoid having to consider taking medicine with its possible side effects to try to improve bone strength. Osteoporosis is preventable in most instances, and by knowing your risk factors and acting in time, you can reduce your risk of painful and life-changing fractures.

General questions to ask yourself:

- What is the picture I see of myself at the future date I have chosen?
- Hunched over and walking slowly, or walking straight up with purpose?
- Do I want to be afraid to go out when it is slippery because I might fall?
- Do I want to get results over the phone telling me my bones are weak?
- Do I want to learn that I could have prevented my weak bones by just taking a supplement and walking 5,000 steps per day?
- Do I have to consider taking medication to keep from having a hip fracture?

More specifically for W*A*I*Pointes™, in which category does your POS fit?

3—Low risk heart	- Activity 30 minutes per day
- Adequate Vitamin D and calcium
- Non-smoker
- Two or fewer alcohol servings per day
- Post menopause and FRAX score (developed in England, it looks at your risk factors for a fracture. Helps you decide if you need medical treatment.) less than 3%
- Pre-menopause: 0-2 risk factors
2—Moderate risk	- Pre-menopause: 3-5 risk factors
- Inadequate activity
- Inconsistent Vitamin D and calcium
- 2 alcohol servings per day
1—High risk	- Post-menopause with prior fragility fracture
- Hip or vertebral fracture
- FRAX hip >3% or total >20%
- Pre-menopause 5+ risk factors

H. Heart Disease

With heart disease being the number one killer of women, it is the culprit that is most likely to shorten your life. Heart disease can also progressively limit your quality of life by keeping you from doing what you want to do. Many women have to take several medicines every day to slow down the disease process, reduce the chance of a heart attack and/or stroke, and to maintain their daily activities. Heart disease can be silent, but we know what risk factors to look for and ways to test for the disease.

This preventable illness causes shortness of breath, fatigue, difficulty exercising, leg pain, and strokes. It is caused by the inflammation and deposit of blood cholesterol in the blood vessel walls. Heart disease can start very early depending on the number of risk factors a woman has including obesity, high blood pressure, high blood sugars (with pre-diabetes and diabetes), and high cholesterol. Women are at higher risk of developing heart disease if they are inactive, have Polycystic Ovarian Syndrome, or have had toxemia or pre-eclampsia/eclampsia during pregnancy.

It is well known that heart disease is prevented by living a heart-healthy lifestyle including regular exercise, a diet low in saturated fat and sugar, and by maintaining a healthy weight. For women with a high risk of developing heart disease as a result of their family history and genetics, or because of years of bad habits, even small improvements in activity level and weight loss can prolong their life. Medicines that lower cholesterol and blood pressure, and treat diabetes can delay a heart attack and stroke by many years and improve quality of life. By looking at my own personal risk factors, I would probably have a heart attack at the age of 150. But, if I fall off the health wagon and gain weight, let my cholesterol go up, or start eating more sugar and develop pre-diabetes, I could speed up the inevitable and make my heart attack happen earlier.

In the concept of W*A*I*Pointes™, I want you to think about heart disease in the same way you think about your financial retirement plans. Think about how long you want to live. How do you want to function while you are living? Most of us do not think about how clean our blood vessels are on a daily basis, but by the time we have shortness of breath or exercise-induced fatigue, the vessels are already thickened or blocked.

A heart-healthy lifestyle includes daily activity of 30 minutes or more, not smoking, not being exposed to secondhand smoke, and maintaining a healthy weight. The risk factors (which can be made better or worse by lifestyle and medicines) include Body Mass Index (BMI); waist circumference; blood pressure; C-reactive protein (a measurement of body inflammation); blood levels of triglycerides, HDL-cholesterol, LDL-cholesterol, total cholesterol, blood sugars, and HgA1C (a measurement of average blood sugar levels over a three month period).

In defining your POS, I want you to think about her not only in terms of what she can do, but also objectively with numbers as they correlate to specific risk factors. One way to determine your risk is with the Reynolds Risk Score. It is designed to help you predict your risk of having a future heart attack, stroke, or other major heart disease within the next 10 years. You can decide how "good" you want your score to be. The scoring process can be found at reynoldsriskscore.org. The trick is to learn how to get your current state to match up with your POS. In future chapters, we will help you with that.

General questions to ask yourself:

- Does my POS have a healthy heart and clean blood vessels?
- Is my heart as healthy as it could be? Is it healthy and strong, or slow and weak?

- Are my blood vessels clean and smooth, or is there clogging plaque and sticky walls? Can I exercise without stopping to catch my breath?
- Can I go for a walk without having to limit the distance?
- Can I hike the park, or do I have to stop and walk because of fatigue or shortness of breath?
- Should my POS be prepared to call 911 or go to the Emergency Room for chest pain? Does my POS take heart medications?

More specifically for W*A*I*Pointes™, in which category does your POS fit?

3—Low risk heart attack	<ul><li>Reynolds score <5%</li><li>Heart healthy lifestyle</li><li>No smoking</li><li>Healthy diet with ≤2 red meat per week</li><li>Physically active</li><li>BMI ≤30</li><li>≤7 alcohol per week</li></ul>
2—Moderate risk heart attack	<ul><li>Reynolds score 5-20%</li><li>Inactivity (≤150 min. per week)</li><li>BMI ≥30</li><li>Waist circumference ≥35"</li><li>FH premature CAD</li><li>High blood pressure controlled</li><li>High LDL or low HDL cholesterol or high triglycerides</li><li>Metabolic syndrome</li></ul>

| | - Poor exercise capacity
- Hx of pre-eclampsia
- Gestational diabetes
- PCOS |
|---|---|
| 1—High risk heart attack | - Reynolds score >20%
- Diagnosed coronary heart disease (microvascular or luminal)
- PAD
- CVD
- High blood pressure not controlled
- Undiagnosed chest pain or shortness of breath |

I. Income Security:

Income security is a challenging question. For many, income is not so secure and there is daily stress to make ends meet. For some, there is secure income but because of fear, or poor planning, there still does not seem to ever be enough money. Studies have shown that happiness does not improve with more money, beyond our ability to pay our basic bills and save something for the future, but unhappiness is associated with worry of not having enough for bills. Some women may choose to stay in unhealthy relationships because of money, and many lie awake at night with worry. And, many of us, including myself, were not taught how to handle money, and were aware at a young age that money was a concern for the family. Fear and not knowing can be a difficult barrier to overcome. So, it is time to face the black and white numbers on paper or a screen and decide how you want to be in the future.

As you look through how to classify your POS in the future, you will see that it is not just about how much money you have, but about being honest and clear about: what resources you have, your safety net, and living within your means. Facing money fears and asking these questions can be the most important steps in reducing stress about money and on the way to total mind and body wellness.

General questions to ask yourself:

- How is my POS and her relationship with money?
- Is it fear-based or am I confident, at least knowing the facts and spending what I have?
- Does my POS know my financial picture?
- Am I dependent on other people for income and meeting basic needs?
- Do I want to toss and turn at night worrying about money?
- Are my financial books orderly and balanced?
- Do I have a safety net to pay my bills if I lose my income?
- Will I be able to retire and pay my bills, as well as enjoy life?
- Will I have to choose one medication over the other because I cannot afford both?
- Does my POS get to leave a legacy of financial smarts as well as financial gifts for my loved ones? Or is my POS going to leave bills for others to pay?

More specifically for W*A*I*Pointes™, in which category does your POS fit?

3—Low Risk	
	• Future secured
	• Savings plan in place
	• Safety net of at least three months expenses
	• Budget in place and followed

2—Moderate Risk	- No future plan in place or no professional review
- Safety net of three or less months worth of expenses
- Bills paid with budget in place
- Low or no credit card balances
1—High Risk	- No future plans or savings
- No security net
- Budget not in place
- Some bills go unpaid
- High credit card balances and usage

Take the score for each of these categories and plot them on the Life Action Plan in the W*A*I*Pointes™ workbook (available at truewomenshealth.com). Add for a total score.

Summary

Sometimes when I sit at a bookstore drinking my soy-milk cappuccino, I look at other people's food and drink choices. Time and again, I see the food choices match the body type. I remember seeing a couple of retirement age, obese and moving slowly, eating their cream soup and drinking their caramel whole milk lattes. Do they know that the same pleasures can be had in healthy versions of the same foods and smaller portions, and taste much better when the treat or meal follows a brisk walk? Do they know healthy choices would allow them to sit in the bleachers when watching their grandchildren play basketball?

Once we understand what it is we want, and develop that picture, we will have a goal to work toward. First we need to be free to write our thoughts of that person we want to become. Let us develop the idea of the image: physically, mentally, and spiritually. Let us think in color and pay attention to the tiniest of details. Start here, and start now.

The rest of this book is about how to reach your POS. In some areas you might decide to settle for a higher weight than you originally thought, or a less aggressive activity goal, depending on what is realistic for your lifestyle and current situation. And, as you get more comfortable with this process, you can adjust over time as you see fit and are able. But, no matter your POS, you are on a path of always moving forward.

My Personal Picture of Self (POS): Dr. Diana L. Bitner

Now that I am 48, my POS is me at age 53. That's when my youngest child will be graduating from high school. I imagine myself excited and happy at the graduation party, my mind racing with memories, hopes, and dreams, wanting my son to have an abundant and full life.

In my POS, I'm healthy and strong, fit and looking fabulous, smiling at my husband, proud to be hosting such an event. As well as a mom and wife, I want to be working to pursue my vision of improving women's health and the health care system. I want to be without regrets, not the woman who says, "If only I was more active," or "If only I had not eaten all that junk," or "If only I had taken my Vitamin D!"

I want to be doing sit-ups and boy-pushups and be able to walk up a flight of stairs when I am 70. So, just like everyone else, I need to be clear about my future self and plan for my future.

My POS is as follows:

A. Activity

No bunions, no hip pain, and no tight muscles to limit me or ache at night. No barriers I cannot get around. Able to ski, run, Jet Ski, run in a 5K with my kids, jump around a sailboat, go into a water park with my grandkids and go down the slides with them—not watch them, but ride with them. Ride horses on the beach in Ireland. Hike mountains in Appalachia. Bike all over Mackinac Island with my husband. Be active without pain or fear!

B. Obesity

Weight: 125 lbs. or so, waist less than 35 inches, body fat percentage under 25. My POS has a great mantra: "Lean and ease of movement" and she does not like anything to slow her down.

C. Cancer

Hell no! I have too much to give and do. I do not want to be scared like that and I never want to hear the "C" word. I want to be around a long time with my kids. My POS is doing everything she can to avoid cancer of the breast, lung, or colon; therefore, she is at a healthy weight, drinks minimal alcohol and eats only rare saturated fat in her diet. She does not smoke and is not exposed to secondhand smoke.

D. Diabetes

I do not want to have diabetes or be insulin resistant. I do not want to have sugar cravings and do not want to have to poke my finger for blood sugar readings. I am a wimp when it comes to pain. Therefore, I am aware of my portion sizes and take little bites; I am aware of what choices I need to make, like choosing sweet potatoes instead of white potatoes and the importance of keeping my weight down. If I start to gain weight around my middle, I know it is a red flag warning of the need to scale back on simple carbohydrates like treats or bread or wine.

E. Ease of Coping

Life is hard, and there are always curve balls. People change, the world changes, and bad stuff happens out of our control. We cannot control others' actions or responses. I want to maintain my positive outlook, ask for help when needed, and remember what is important, how to be true to myself, and how I want to live my life with peace, love, calm and truth. I want to maintain my way of coping with lists, big picture planning, find a community to be around me and be able to communicate.

F. Phase of Ovarian Function

I want to know where I am with the hormone thing and keep my estrogen receptors happy. I do not have time for the symptoms of hot flashes, night sweats, or poor sleep. I need to get up refreshed and be ready for surgery, my family, and seeing a day of patients. I want to feel happy and be in a good mood inside and out. I do not want vaginal dryness or unnecessary bladder urgency, and I do not want heavy periods. I want to know what I can do in my lifestyle to feel good through my transition into menopause, as well as what options exist for hormone replacement when the time is right. And, I want to know when the time is right, and if they are safe for me personally.

G. Good Bones

I know bone loss is silent and I do not want to have to worry about breaking bones and not being able to ski or ride horses. As I mentioned, I am a wimp and do not do well with pain; therefore, the thought of micro fractures in my spine freaks me out. I have seen women with this. So, I will be clear with my desire for strong bones and do what I can to keep them this way.

H. Heart Disease

My risk for heart disease is currently low and that is how I want it to stay. I do not want to die of something preventable, or at least have it happen when I am ready to go at age 100. I do not want to be on a bed in the hallway at the ER waiting for my heart tests to come back, or worry that a hike in the mountains could have me ending up with chest pan, or have to stop because of it. I want to be able to keep up with my friends or kids on a hike.

I. Income Security

I cannot stand to worry about money. This goes back to being a child and watching my parents go through a divorce and feeling uncertainty about everything. It extended into college when I worried every year if I was going to be able to return the next year, and in medical school when I could not afford a haircut. I have felt how worrying about finances can be a powerful deterrent from a good night's sleep. So, financial health for my POS means bills are paid, a safety net is in place for at least three months of expenses, and savings for retirement and extra expenses are tucked away. At 53, I want to be able to help support my children in college, be able to visit them when I want, and afford to travel and experience other cultures. I also want to be able to donate to college scholarship funds and help to reduce childhood hunger.

In Conclusion: I want to live my life vibrant and strong, without fear, without regret, with minimal medicines and medical problems, and if something bad happens, such as cancer (which I do not want), I can fight it knowing I did everything to prevent it.

Chapter Five

Understanding My Place in Process (PIP)

"Midlife today is a second puberty of sorts. The experience, including its length, is being redefined. It is a period distinctly unlike youth, yet distinctly unlike old age. It doesn't feel like a cruise to the end of our lives so much as a cruise, at last, to the meaning of our lives."

~<u>The Age of Miracles: Embracing the New Midlife</u>
by Marianne Williamson

Now that you have defined your POS, I want to help you move to the next stage toward making your POS happen. That's where Place in Process (PIP) comes in. Think of PIP as a health inventory or an assessment of where you are now, like a snapshot in time. Another way to think about this process is to continue the analogy of a retirement savings plan.

Picture yourself back in front of a financial planner. You say, "I want to retire at 64 with $1,000,000 in savings." The financial planner says, "Okay, how much do you have saved now? And, what are your money habits? How much money is coming in and how much is going out?" The PIP is the same as taking a picture of your health status right now to determine how far off you are from your goal—your POS. Once we know the gap, you can decide to either change your goal to be closer to your PIP, or get busy learning how to close the gap in time to achieve your POS by your goal date or event.

Perimenopause can be a time where the PIP goes downhill to the point where we know we need help, but we don't know where to start or who to turn to. Do night sweats and middle of the night bathroom breaks prevent you from getting the sleep you crave? Do you remember what it was like to wake up feeling rested and energetic? Are you juggling the demands of caring for an aging parent and on-the-go teenagers? Are you noticing your stomach starting to pooch out? Is it starting to look and feel like an inner tube that could keep you afloat in a pool?

This baseline assessment will help you jumpstart simple shifts that will restore the equilibrium to your constantly changing world. It will help you transition to a lifetime ahead of good health. I am here to help put you back in the driver's seat, and help you put your health and wellness back on the priority list in a practical way so you can still take care of others as you wish to do. I am here at your side as guide, coach and sorority sister. We're all in this together.

How to Map Your Journey

From the questions in each category, you will be able to chart your PIP and compare it to your POS. It will give you a freeze-frame view of where you are positioned and what needs to be done in terms of health success. You can then determine if you want to make the changes that will make all the difference. We will use the W*A*I*Pointes™ Wellness categories you have become familiar with. Only this time, instead of using them to visualize what can be, I am asking you to identify what is and where are you today.

This will give you and your doctor, nurse practitioner, or nurse midwife a framework and tools to help you live out your dreams. Your health will support you instead of stand in your way. I challenge you to ask yourself a series of questions in each category of

W*A*I*Pointes™. Also, reference the workbook to really do the work (available at truewomenshealth.com). I think you will be amazed at the freedom you will get from knowing where to focus your efforts and the sense of power which will come from understanding why you feel the way you do.

Back to the Future

If you could look into your future and get a glimpse of the negative impact of not taking care of yourself—be it heart attack or stroke, diabetes or cancer—wouldn't you be scared straight? Would you then choose a different path? Once women understand how preventable illnesses impact everyday life, I believe they will take charge of their own health. I believe women will initiate small changes that will make a big difference.

The PIP process helps you appreciate where you are in all areas of living, from risk for cardiac disease to risk for obesity and cancer. It's also important to know how you cope with stressful situations, similar to your financial situation. All these factors are crucial in being able to focus on making healthy choices. We also need to examine our daily choices, such as "What do I eat every day?"

When you chart your place on the PIP, you are assessing your wellness and then matching it with your emotions, spiritual self and whole self. You will know where you are, where you want to go, and we will figure out together what you need to do to get there. The plan works with you as an individual. The critical component is for you to commit to where you want to be at the age you choose and then compare it to now. Since the idea of wellness is overwhelming, I broke it down in parts. From my experience both personally and professionally with my patients, I saw critical areas that cover most of the aspects of our lives.

In each area, there are ways to consistently judge ability and to assess risk factors for certain illnesses and diseases that can limit our capability and wellness. By assessing where you are now, you create a system to tell if you are improving or not, and if you have reached a plateau.

Are you ready to assess your current state of health and wellbeing? Let's do it!

A. Ability to be Active

To assess your ability to be active, first think about how active you are now, compared with how active you see yourself at the date or event of your POS. If you want to be running a 5K, are you doing that now? If you are gardening and have a lush vegetable or flower garden in your POS, are you currently able to lift, bend and get low to the ground in order to plant that garden? And if you want to be able to ride a bike around your neighborhood or walk a 5K breast cancer walk, are you able to do all of that now?

To be more specific for the W*A*I*Pointes™ category, there are measurements you need to get. First there is a fitness test to take. It is just like the Presidential Fitness Test we took when we were kids in gym class; it turns out there is one for adults as well. To take the test, go to adultfitnesstest.org and sign up. You might need help with recording your results, or at least to have a friend cheering you on.

You will be tested on:
- how long it takes you to run or walk a mile
- how far you can stretch, and
- several basic measurements of strength.

No, you do not have to climb a rope hanging from a ceiling. Once you input the results, it will tell you how you compare with other women your age and give you a percentile result. Write that information in the workbook. Then look over your schedule from the last several weeks and look at how many minutes you spent in aerobic activity where you got your heart rate up, and also how many strength training events you do each week. Record these in the workbook as well.

The next step is to think about the barriers that can derail you from exercise. For example, many of my patients talk about the fact they feel they have no time, no energy, or no money to belong to an exercise club or gym. The barriers can be physical limitations such as chronic back pain, bunions, a surgery you have not recovered from yet, or lack of knowledge about what to do. There are many barriers people experience; now is the time to be honest and name yours. We all know that the first step to finding a solution is to name the problem. List your barriers in the workbook.

3—Very Active Presidential Fitness Score >66 percentile (66%)	<ul><li>More fit than 66% of women your age</li><li>Doing more than 10,000 steps per day or more than 110 minutes of aerobic activity per week</li><li>Strength training more than 3x per week</li><li>Only the rare barrier keeps you from your plan</li></ul>
2—Moderately Active Presidential Fitness Score >33 percentile (33%)	<ul><li>More fit than 33% of women your age</li><li>Moving between 5,000 and 10,000 steps per day</li><li>Strength training 0-2x per week</li><li>1-3 barriers that could derail you from your plan any day</li></ul>

1—Limited activity Presidential Fitness Score <33 percentile (33%)	• Less fit than 33% of women your age • Moving less than 5,000 steps per day • No strength training event per week • 3 or more barriers to activity exist which daily disrupt your chances of activity

2. Obesity

The word Obesity here defines the category about weight. I talk about weight as a wellness category—although it is not the only defining factor of wellness. We do not all have to be skinny to be happy and healthy, but at a weight where we feel good and are healthy. To figure out your PIP, first think about your obesity category for your POS—your weight, your waist circumference, and your body fat percentage. What did you decide you wanted as your POS? Are you already at your POS guidelines or on a path to meeting them? What do you think your PIP is in comparison to your POS? We will use the same three groupings that we used for POS.

So, you need to get your measurements. First, you need to weigh yourself, preferably without any clothes on, or at least in the same clothing items you will weigh yourself each time. Then access a BMI (Body Mass Index) chart at your doctor's office—you can either call your doctor's medical assistant or ask the front office staff to look up your weight and height and give you a BMI measurement, or use an online BMI chart to determine your BMI. Record these numbers in the workbook (available on the website at truewomenshealth.com).

Next, get a tape measure and measure your waist circumference. Feel your hip bones in the front, and starting at the level of the small of your back, bring the tape measure around in front. Record your number.

The last measurement we need is harder to get; however, you should be able to access one at your doctor's office, local health club, or the YMCA. I have an impedance scale in my office; it measures body fat percentage by sending a weak electrical current through your body. Depending on your fat percentage, the speed of the current traveling around your body and back into the scale differs, and gives an indirect measure of your fat percentage, or conversely, your lean body mass. W*A*I*Pointes™ uses these measurements to come up with a grouping which infers more or less risk to your wellness.

3—Healthy	• Waist circumference <35 inches • BMI <25.0 • Body fat percentage in healthy range for your age (20-40: 21-33%, 41-60: 23-35%, and 61-79: 24-36%)
2—Overweight	• Waist circumference between 35-39 inches • BMI between 25-29.9 • Body fat percentage in overweight range (20-40: 33-39%, 41-60: 35-40%, 61-79: 36-42%)

1—Obese	• Waist circumference 40 inches • BMI >30 • Body fat percentage obese (20-40: >39%, 41-60: >40%, 61-79: >42%)

3. Cancer

Cancer steals time, energy, and wellness away from too many lives. Therefore, it is time to figure out your personal risk factors and do what you can to make a difference according to your POS. Cancer occurs because of genetics, environment, and for other reasons we do not know. However, based on well-known risk factors, there are things you can do to lower your risk. And, if you know what to do, I like to think you could help your family and friends do the same. These W*A*I*Pointes™ groupings of risk categories were put together based on recognized risk factors and validated scales of risk. By putting these categories in the program, and in the hands of real people on a widespread basis, we will learn which risk factors are most important, which behaviors matter most, and how modifying your behaviors (such as eating healthier and adding exercise) will potentially reduce cancer risk. No other program exists like W*A*I*Pointes™ to allow you to define your wellness and clearly see what changes might be effective to bring you closer to your dreams.

The references used in this wellness category were derived from a publicly available scale on the Washington University website and the Gale model for breast cancer risk. I mention these for transparency, and in no way intend to claim ownership to their work of validating risk factor scales.

To determine your PIP for cancer, we start with lung cancer. If it is easier for you, go directly to the workbook and fill out the chart. If you have a diagnosis of cancer, you are in the high risk category and no behavior will lower your risk, but staying in the high risk category is better than the alternative! We focus on changing what we can, and focusing on supporting your health in every other area to reduce the chance of the cancer ever coming back.

To determine your risk, you will have to look at your family history (FH), your lifestyle habits, where you live, whether the dirt that your house or apartment is built on contains radon, and your physical statistics. The information requested includes: smoking history; work history; whether you live near a big city; FH of lung, breast, or colorectal cancer; and whether they were pre- or postmenopausal when they were diagnosed with the cancer. If you received high dose radiation in your life for another cancer, such as lymphoma or other medical conditions, it is a risk factor for future cancer. Also your symptoms matter—whether you have chest pain, shortness of breath, any blood in the mucus you cough up, or unexplained weight loss. For colorectal cancer there are more questions about lifestyle habits, including amount of alcohol you take in per day, how much red meat you consume, your level of activity, and your vitamin intake. It is also important to know how often, and when, you received colorectal cancer screening. For breast cancer, many of the same lifestyle questions apply, including activity, alcohol consumption, as well as physical characteristics such as genetic history and BMI.

Later in the book, we will look at ways to improve your PIP to match your POS by the date or event to which you have committed. First, we have to know where you stand today.

Types/Cancer	Lung	Colorectal	Breast
3—Low Risk	No smoking ever; Former, quit ≥20 yrs ago	≥50 yrs, normal colonoscopy; ≤3 srvgs red meat/week; ≤1 alcohol/day; Vit D & calcium; ≥30 min exercise most days	No 1st degree relative pre-menopause breast cancer; No prior biopsies; ≥30 min exercise/day; ≤1 alcohol/day; BMI ≤30; Screening
2—Moderate Risk	Quit ≤20 yrs; Large city 10+ yrs; Long secondhand smoke; Factory wk. ≥10 yrs; Radiation exposure	Hx of colon polyps; Family hx of lg polyps; IBS ≥10 yrs; ≥2 red meat/wk; ≥1 alcohol/day; No screening colonoscopy	Family hx 1st degree post-menopause breast cancer; ≤30 min exercise/day; 1-2 alcohol/day; BMI ≥30
1—High Risk	Current smoker; Prior lung cancer; High risk symptoms: changing cough, shortness breath, chest pain, cough up blood	Personal hx colon cancer; 1st degree relative colon cancer; Family cancer syndromes; Symptoms: blood in stool, change in BM, chronic abdominal pain	Family hx 1st degree relative pre-menopause breast cancer; FH male breast cancer; BRCA 1 or 2+; prior breast cancer; Past high dose radiation; Gale ≥20%

4. Diabetes

Diabetes is a disease process in which there is a viscous cycle of insulin resistance (the cells do not listen to insulin and open up as they should to receive sugar), high blood sugars and higher than normal insulin production. At some point in the process, the body cannot make enough insulin, and blood sugars are so high that taking insulin is required to avoid dangerous levels, true sugar coma, etc. Over time, high blood sugar levels can damage small blood vessels in the eyes, brain, toes, and clitoris/penis leading to stroke, blindness, and sexual dysfunction. Early in the process, when it is still at the level of prediabetes, type 2 diabetes can be prevented. Type 2 diabetes itself can be managed and sugars kept in control, but once it is diagnosed, there are health risks which are not easily reversed. So, let's figure out where you are in your process—your PIP!

3—Low Risk	<ul><li>No family hx of type 2 diabetes</li><li>Normal fasting blood sugar and glucose tolerance</li><li>Waist circumference <35 inches</li></ul>
2—Moderate Risk	<ul><li>Impaired fasting blood sugar</li><li>Hx of PCOS (polycystic ovarian syndrome)</li><li>Hx of metabolic syndrome</li><li>Hx of gestational diabetes</li><li>Family hx of type 2 diabetes</li><li>Waist circumference >35 inches</li></ul>

	• Symptoms of sugar craving and easy weight gain
1—High Risk	• Hx of type 2 diabetes • Fasting blood sugar >125 mg/dl • HgA1C > 6.5% • Random blood sugar > 200 mg/dl

Abbreviations:

FH: family history
FBS: fasting blood sugar
GTT: glucose tolerance test,
HgA1C: hemoglobin % with sugar, measures sugar levels over 3 months
PCOS: polycystic ovarian syndrome
GDM: gestational diabetes
DM: diabetes mellitus

Write your answers in your workbook, and be able to chart your way forward! If you are a 3, great—let us figure out how to maintain that. If you are a 2, you can choose to return your numbers to a 3, or maintain at a 2. If you are a 1, you have many choices as well—to maintain other areas of wellness to lower your risk of heart disease, or return to a 2. We are here to help. What is your PIP?

5. Ease of Coping

It is important to know how well you cope in certain situations. In W*A*I*Pointes™ we use a validated scale to understand your depressive symptoms, your anxiety symptoms, and the Brief Cope Scale, which was invented by CS Carver at the University of Miami. This was not validated in women in midlife or menopause, and no scoring system is available. He has given permission for the scale to be used (see his website listed below), and we plan to validate it so we understand better how to apply the results. For the time being, we have to be creative and start by bringing up the topic, and work to understand how our ability to cope with stress and life situations affects our health and wellness. For now, therefore, the PIP scale is as follows:

3—Resilient–low risk for poor coping	• PHQ-9 0-4 • Habit of maintaining a positive outlook • Honest with self and others • Established support group
2—Moderate risk for adequate coping	• PHQ-9 5-14 • Currently lost positive outlook • Increased anxiety • Some dysfunction in relationships or work because of coping methods • Lost contact with support group, but they exist

1—High risk for poor coping	• PHQ-9 15-27 • Not able to keep positive outlook • Depression or anxiety crippling relationships or work • No support group

To better understand yourself, go to the websites listed below and take the Brief Cope Scale. A higher score is better with a max of 48 points for really good coping skills. Then take the PHQ-9 and score yourself. Make a list of the people you could call in an emergency or just to talk and get support. Be honest with yourself, would you and do you call on other people when you are having a hard time?

To fill out your workbook, first think about your outlook. Can you see that all is going to be okay and you believe you will be fine? Can you list off several people you trust who you could, and would, be willing to call if you needed to talk, vent, or check your thinking about an event that stressed you out? Do you believe you deserve a good life and are you able to think clearly and make plans to overcome barriers that come your way? Then you are a 3.

If you score a 2, you could go either way depending on your stress level, your health, your situation, and the amount of stress which presents itself.

If you score a 1, you are at high risk for not coping well, which could lead to yet worse outcomes; a breakdown in your relationships and work, and affect your health in a bad way. It is time to get help, starting with your health care provider and should involve counseling. Think of anyone in your life you can trust and lean on them now! In better times, you can be there for them!

Brief COPE www.psy.miami.edu/faculty/ccarver/sclBrCOPE.html
PHQ-9--
http://www.integration.samhsa.gov/images/res/PHQ%20-%20Questions.pdfhttp://www.med.umich.edu/1info/FHP/practiceguides/depress/score.pdf

6. Phase of Ovarian Function

The first step in determining your PIP in the Phase of Ovarian Function wellness category is to know where you are in the process. I used the STRAW Diagram (Stages of Ovarian Aging Workshop) information in 2011 to make a flowchart which will allow you to use the information to determine where you are in the stages of ovarian aging. By knowing where you are, you will know more of what to expect.

To determine your PIP, there is information you will need to know:

- the date of your last period
- the longest period of time between periods, and
- the basic schedule of your periods over the last year or so.

If you have had a hysterectomy but still have your ovaries, obviously you will not have had a period, and therefore will have to go by any cyclical symptoms like mood change, headaches, night sweats, and hot flashes. These symptoms are more likely to occur in the few days before your period would have started, if you still had your uterus. Also, your menopause doctor could order a blood test called FSH (follicle stimulating hormone). One blood level measurement does not tell your story, but especially if you have had a hysterectomy, the level can give clues depending on when in your cycle it was drawn.

Dr. Diana L. Bitner, MD, NCMP

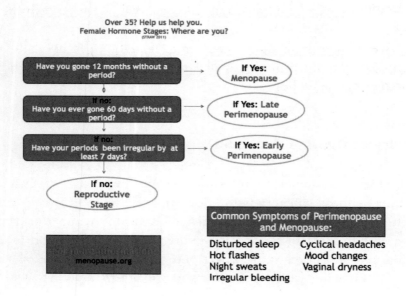

Many women return to the health care system because of these symptoms, which can be very confusing and interfere with quality of life in a powerful way. These symptoms are very treatable, even without medications. Simple factor such as hydration, body weight, diet, sleep, and stress levels affect these symptoms. By understanding which symptoms you are having, we can determine how to best get you feeling better. Knowing where you rank in the category can help us track your progress over time to determine which treatments are working and which are not.

Your PIP is determined by whether or not you know your phase, and the degree of bother you are experiencing from your symptoms related to midlife and menopause. In the two weeks prior to taking this MTS quiz (see page 120), what symptoms have you experienced at the level described in the MTS (Chapter Seven)?

Fill out the chart in the workbook, and we will compare your PIP to your POS and chart on the Life Action Plan in a later chapter. MTS is as below:

To create your PIP score, there are 3 categories:

3—Minimal/predictable functional	<ul><li>Minimal or rare distress: no or rare hormone related symptoms</li><li>MTS >19</li><li>Knowledge of phase and symptoms</li></ul>
2—Moderate distress with some effect on daily life	<ul><li>Symptoms mild and predictable</li><li>MTS 12-18</li></ul>
1—Low quality of life-dysfunctional	<ul><li>Able to sometimes predict symptoms and severe distress</li><li>MTS <12</li><li>Minimal knowledge of symptoms triggers, no knowledge of phases.</li></ul>

If your PIP does not match up to your POS, or how you want to be, then it is time to look at options for feeling better. See Chapter Six for a list of options.

7. Good bones – Osteoporosis and risk of fracture and pain

To understand what support or actions are to be taken to make sure your bones are as strong and healthy as you wish them to be, we must look at risk factors for bone loss. Bone loss is silent. There are normal rates of bone loss as we age, with an expected acceleration when we lose our estrogen through natural or surgical menopause. When the loss is greater than expected, there can be other causes such as Vitamin D deficiency, excess phosphate soda in our diet, or medical conditions such as multiple myeloma or hyperparathyroidism. To determine your PIP, we will score based on these factors:

3—Low Risk	<ul><li>Activity 30 minutes per day</li><li>Adequate Vitamin D and calcium</li><li>Non-smoker</li><li>Two or fewer alcohol servings per day</li><li>Post-menopause and FRAX score (Developed in England, it looks at your risk factors for a fracture. Helps you decide if you need medical treatment.) less than 3%</li><li>Pre-menopause 0-2 risk factors</li></ul>
2—Moderate Risk	<ul><li>Pre-menopause 3-5 risk factors</li><li>Inadequate activity</li><li>Inconsistent Vitamin D and calcium</li><li>2 alcohol servings per day</li></ul>

1—High Risk	• Post-menopause with prior fragility fracture • Hip or vertebral fracture • FRAX hip >3% or total >20% • Pre-menopause 5+ risk factors

8. Heart disease

To determine your PIP for heart disease, we use a female-specific risk scoring system which is validated and available to the public, as well as the well-known risk factor of metabolic syndrome and other factors. Heart disease is preventable, or at least able to be delayed. This risk system will inform you of your level of risk for having a heart attack, or at least being limited by chest pain and shortness of breath and will help inform you about the options you have to reduce your risk as you wish.

The Reynolds Score is available at reynoldsriskscore.org and was developed to help doctors understand more about heart disease risk. Using the Framingham Risk Score for heart disease in women, leaves many women in the intermediate category. This has made it difficult to know how best to treat women in this category in terms of who needs aggressive treatment, including medications, and who does not. The intent of the authors of the Reynolds Score was to determine which of the women in the intermediate category of Framingham are truly at enough risk for a heart attack to warrant aggressive treatment. It has been shown to be successful at improving understanding of women's heart disease risk, as it is different than men's heart disease.

3—Low risk heart attack	- Reynolds score <5% - Heart healthy lifestyle - No smoking - Healthy diet with ≤2 red meat per week - Physically active - BMI ≤30 - ≤7 alcohol per week
2—Moderate risk heart attack	- Reynolds score 5-20% - Inactivity (≤150 min. per week) - BMI ≥30 - Waist circumference ≥35" - FH premature CAD - High blood pressure controlled - High LDL or low HDL cholesterol or high triglycerides - Metabolic syndrome - Poor exercise capacity - Hx of pre-eclampsia - Gestational diabetes - PCOS
1—High risk heart attack	- Reynolds score >20% - Diagnosed coronary heart disease (microvascular or luminal) - PAD - CVD - High blood pressure not controlled - Undiagnosed chest pain or shortness of breath

9. Income Security

In order for you to reach your financial security goals, it is necessary to know how much you have, to face your financial habits of saving and spending, and face the fear many of us have about not having enough. Studies show that excess money does not buy happiness, but not having enough to provide basic security and care for our dependents is linked to happiness.

There are well know determinants of financial security, and the PIP score is based on these basics. Again, Income Security is not about having excess money, this wellness category is about going over the basics and making sure the three main bases are covered to provide peace of mind and security.

3—Low Risk	<ul><li>Future secured</li><li>Savings plan in place</li><li>Safety net of at least three months expenses</li><li>Budget in place and followed</li></ul>
2—Moderate Risk	<ul><li>No future plan in place or no professional review</li><li>Safety net of three or less months worth of expenses</li><li>Bills paid with budget in place</li><li>Low or no credit card balances</li></ul>
1—High Risk	<ul><li>No future plans or savings</li><li>No security net</li></ul>

	<ul><li>Budget not in place</li><li>Some bills go unpaid</li><li>High credit card balances and usage</li></ul>

Chapter Six

Feeling Better Using SEEDS™

"Unrelieved stress affects almost every function of the body, causing insomnia, high blood pressure, constipation, depression and an assortment of anxiety-driven aches and pains."

~Pamela Peeke, MD, author of <u>Fight Fat after Forty</u> and <u>Body for Life for Women: A Woman's Plan for Physical and Mental Transformation</u>

Are you ready to stop waiting for the 'change' and start making the lifestyle changes that will move you with grace, joy and energy into your 50s and beyond? Let's get going.

The first step to alleviating the uncomfortable physical changes of midlife is to identify which symptoms you are experiencing—irritability, hot flashes, sleep disturbance—and track when they happen. Once you recognize what is going on in your body and pay attention to what's happening when these symptoms surface, you'll be able to pinpoint what behaviors or daily habits may be making them worse. And then you can choose what to do.

For example, what would you rather have, that third cup of coffee which will trigger a mid-afternoon hot flash; or water, an apple and a cheese stick? That second glass of wine and resulting night sweats or an extra glass of water and a good night's sleep? Studies show that decreasing caffeine and alcohol intake while increasing water intake and activity level will help decrease the severity or frequency of hot flashes. The point is that implementing incremental changes in your daily life will make a difference.

We need to recognize that our bodies have non-negotiable needs to function well optimally. These essential elements are not optional and when we ignore or deny these necessities, we impact our well-being and quality of life. I've dubbed these non-negotiables SEEDS™, an acronym for Seven Essential Elements for Daily Success. These essentials are: water, sleep, micronutrients (vitamins), macronutrients (food groups), fiber, activity and mind/body wellness. I have had many patients just start doing their SEEDS™, nothing else, and they feel much better.

What is SEEDS™?

Seven Essential Elements for Daily Success

SEEDS™
Water/Fluids
Sleep
Micronutrients
Macronutrients
Fiber
Activity
Mind/Body

These seven essentials impact our midlife transition and correlate with success. Bottom line: supply these and you will have good quality of life. There is no magic bullet; it is all about the basic essentials.

We hope that by encouraging you to meet your daily SEEDS™ recommendations, you will successfully improve your overall quality of life.

Seven Essential Elements for Daily Success

1. Water/Fluids—Don't Go Without It

There is controversy on exactly how much water we need, but most of us know what is right for our bodies and activity levels. Are you dizzy and fatigued? Try more water and see what happens!

You need at least six to eight ten-ounce glasses of non-caffeinated beverages per day. Water is the body's principal chemical compound, making up, on average, 60% of a woman's body weight. Nearly every system in your body depends on water. It flushes toxins out of your vital organs, carries nutrients and oxygen to your cells, and helps dissolve nutrients so they are accessible to your body. Water moistens ear, nose and throat tissues. Inadequate water intake causes dehydration, a condition that occurs when you don't have enough water in your body to carry out your normal functions.

Even mild dehydration can cause headache and lethargy. It is well known by athletic trainers that if athletes are not well hydrated, they do not perform as well—they are not as fast, do not have the necessary stamina, and will not win. If they are not well hydrated, their core temperature rises faster, and their muscles under perform. If midlife and menopausal women are not well hydrated, we tend to feel more fatigued, are less likely to get through a workout, less likely to even want to start the work-out, and work out with less intensity. Women who are not well hydrated have more hot flashes and night sweats. I have patients that start drinking more water and notice fewer hot flashes and night sweats. Treatment of our most common symptoms does not have to be rocket science. It is often just back to the basics.

To calculate your water intake per day, the important number is total water MINUS each serving of alcohol and caffeine. Both alcohol and caffeine make you excrete out water even if you are mildly dehydrated. I have had this conversation with some of my patients.

"I drink plenty of water, usually four to five glasses per day."

"How much caffeine?" I ask.

"Four cups."

"How much alcohol?"

"One to two glasses of wine each night."

That is five glasses of water, minus four cups of coffees and two glasses of wine; therefore, the net water is negative two servings. While this is not a scientific demonstration, in real life, this net amount of water affects menopause symptoms, energy, and quality of life.

While research supports the protective effects of alcohol in moderation, it's important to understand and weigh the risks versus benefits of moderate alcohol intake and discuss any concerns with your health care provider.

Because alcohol is dehydrating and constricts the blood vessels, for some women—myself included—even one glass of wine with dinner may trigger a hot flash or night sweats.

About a year ago, I was attending a conference in Washington, D.C. At dinner, I had a glass of red wine, something I rarely do (my limit is two glasses per month). I also ate carbs and a sugary dessert. That night, I went to sleep easily, but woke up with a night sweat. The next night, not registering the connection between my noshing and the night sweat, I did the same thing and lo and behold, another hot flash. It was a light bulb moment. I realized that my wine consumption coupled with the extra carbs and sweets, had thrown my system out of whack. For me, the combo is a trigger and now that I know how these particular triggers affect me, I'll be able to weigh the pros and cons and make more informed choices about what I choose to eat and drink.

Caffeine is a central nervous system stimulant which is why it can temporarily alleviate fatigue and increase wakefulness. On the flip side, its stimulant properties can make you jittery and cause sleep problems. And the negative effects tend to increase during perimenopause and menopause. I am not against caffeine; in fact, I really enjoy my mug of coffee in the morning, either as I get the kids ready, or in my car on the way to work. But, if you're experiencing new or increased insomnia, sleep disturbance, anxiety or irritability, rethink your coffee consumption. Maybe not stop it, but balance it with more water consumption.

In addition, caffeine is a diuretic which means that, like alcohol, it can make us dehydrated and lethargic. How often do we reach for coffee, chocolate or a caffeine-laced diet drink to get us over that 3:00 p.m. slump? If you really must have that afternoon coffee, drink at least eight ounces of water first.

2. Sleep—Sleep is everything (50 hours per week)

For your body, sleep is more precious than gold. Humans can't function without it and don't function well when sleep is disrupted. It can be almost impossible to lose weight if you are sleep deprived!

The first step to repairing your sleep is figuring out your sleep patterns. Do you always have sleep trouble or only at certain times of the month, for example, in the three nights before your period? Or if you are in menopause, did your sleeping difficulties just start when your periods stopped? Or is your lack of sleep because you stay up too late trying to get things done around the house? Or is your slumber affected during super stressful times? Do you have trouble falling asleep? Do you fall asleep easily only to awaken in the night unable to get back to sleep? Do you stay up too late, set the alarm for 5:00 a.m. and then hit snooze five times?

Many experts agree we all need approximately 50 hours of sleep per week, meaning a minimum of seven good quality hours per night. There is controversy on the concept of making up sleep or 'sleep banking'. Sleep experts warn that counting on weekend catch up is not a good idea, but catching up can help if needed. It is better to stick to a schedule.

If you snore, are overweight or obese, drift off at work, or if you've actually fallen asleep at your desk or worse, while driving, you should see your doctor. Some women actually carry a gene which leads to narcolepsy (a poor night's sleep resulting in daytime fatigue), which can be successfully treated by a sleep doctor. You may also need to be evaluated for sleep apnea, which can also be treated.

If you have sleep apnea marked by frequent waking and snoring, you should ask your doctor to refer you to a certified sleep specialist and complete a sleep study. Sleep apnea can be made worse by sleep difficulties caused by fluctuating hormones, and sleep apnea can increase your risk of heart disease.

Treatment of sleep disturbances should first focus on improving sleep routine with good sleep hygiene, including establishing a regular sleep schedule; avoiding heavy evening meals; adjusting levels of light, noise, and temperature in the bedroom; and avoiding alcohol, caffeine, and nicotine.

If you wake up often, get out of bed and empty your bladder, drink a glass of water, sit in the kitchen in a not-too-comfortable chair and begin metered breathing (see next page).

Metered Breathing

- Sit comfortably with your arms relaxed and take a deep cleansing breathe.
- Close your mouth, open your eyes and stare at a small object and breathe.
- If your mind wanders, then, without judgment, go back to breathing.
- The goal is five minutes, twice a day.

Once you get practiced, it is a great tool to do even one minute before a meeting, a confrontation, or an important phone call. This practice gets you back in your body and turns off the fight or flight response, and allows the smart parts of your brain to engage.

Metered breathing also allows our body to maintain a wider thermo neutral zone and decrease hot flashes.

As the yogi Baron Baptiste says, "Focusing on one small thing calms the mind." It can also calm the thermostat so it will not be sensitive to slight changes in temperature.

We cannot always change the stress of our environment, but we can change how our body physically responds to the stress. When we get stressed, our brain says, "Stressful situation—must react." Think of how your body reacts to a fire drill. If a fire alarm goes off, your brain will register what the noise means, and then has a job to do—get you moving to avoid the fire. Your adrenal glands release adrenalin to get you into action. Your liver and muscles release sugar to give your muscles energy to move. Your body reacts to avoid danger. If you feel as if fire drills are going off in your world all day long, and you are frequently stressed and overwhelmed, it can be wearing on your overall energy level. Metered breathing and a practice of gratitude can be helpful tools to cope with a stressful life.

Tips to getting a better night's sleep.

- Keep a daily gratitude journal and worry list to externalize your thoughts. Put them down on paper so you can evict them from your brain. Leave them for a time when you do useful problem solving, not wasteful circle thinking.

- Go to bed at the same time. Wake up at the same time. Ideally, your schedule will remain the same every night of the week.

- Get regular exposure to outdoor light or sunlight, preferably in the late afternoon.

- If you wake up in the middle of the night, don't lie there tossing and turning and feeling frustrated. Get up and try metered breathing.

- If hot flashes or night sweats are becoming a more regular thing, do five minutes of metered breathing before bed to settle down the thermostat and reduce hot flashes at night.

3. Micronutrients—daily multivitamin, calcium and Vitamin D

Vitamins and minerals are worth their weight in gold. A daily multivitamin can be beneficial in supplying trace minerals for body function. Calcium is a multipurpose mineral. It plays a role in nerve transmission and muscle function, and is critical to maintaining our teeth and bones, and reducing the risk of developing osteoporosis, a thinning of the bone that accelerates in postmenopausal women. According to The National Institutes of Health, in the first years after menopause, women lose an estimated 3% to 5% of their bone mass, leveling off at 1% per year after age 65.

The recommended daily dose of calcium for women 19 to 51 years of age is 1,000 mg. For women 51 and over, the Food and Nutrition Board at the Institute of Medicine of the National Academies recommends a daily dose of 1,200 to 2,000 mg. Calcium rich foods include yogurt, milk, kale, sardines with bones, cheese, Chinese cabbage and broccoli. Supplements may be needed for those who are lactose intolerant or can't get the recommended dosage from food sources.

Vitamin D and calcium are like a happily married couple; one doesn't do well without the other. Vitamin D is essential for calcium absorption. Recent research suggests that Vitamin D also plays an important role in the prevention and possible treatment of diseases such as cancer, high blood pressure, diabetes and multiple sclerosis.

The best source of Vitamin D is direct exposure to sunlight. About 10 to 15 minutes of sunlight a day during afternoon hours, three times a week, may be adequate. Other sources of Vitamin D include milk, eggs, fish and cheese. Of the supplements available, Vitamin D3 is most readily absorbed by the body.

How much Vitamin D do you need? A blood test that measures Vitamin D levels is helpful to know if you are deficient and how severely. Emerging research suggests that we need more Vitamin D than the 400 IU recommended daily. If you are significantly overweight, you may need a higher dose.

4. Macronutrients—Carbs, Protein and Fats

Smart eating for energy includes five servings of carbohydrates daily, five servings of proteins and three servings of fats. Here's the skinny on what you need and why you need it.

Carbohydrates: Why do distance runners "carb up" and eat lots of pasta before a marathon? The body needs carbohydrates to make energy. There are two different types of carbohydrates: sugars (or simple carbs) and complex carbs. Smart (good) sources of simple carbs are fruits and dairy. Unhealthy simple carbs include processed sugar such as table sugar, candy, sugary sodas, baked goods and syrups. These are the ones that make us gain weight easily and turn into fat, which is stored in our belly.

Smart (good) sources of complex carbs include vegetables, whole grain breads and pasta, brown rice, oatmeal, and whole grain pastas. Avoid white bread, cakes, cookies, pies, white rice; simple carbs lead to blood sugar highs and lows.

The concept is based on the glycemic index. It is a rating scale based on how fast the carbohydrate is broken down into sugar, how high the sugar spikes in your blood, and how fast your blood sugar then drops. A high glycemic index food is a peppermint candy or orange juice. A low glycemic food is a sweet potato or grapefruit juice. Think how differently you feel after choosing the high glycemic food choice instead of the low glycemic food. If you are paying attention, the low glycemic food has minimal sugar buzz (meaning no brown sugar on your sweet potato) and leaves you feeling full longer. Simple sugars are high glycemic index choices and can trigger a hot flash, or if eaten before bed can trigger a night sweat.

What should your daily serving of carbs be? It is recommended you get 45% to 65% of your calories from carbs. If you are on an 1,800 calorie per day diet, you should eat between 200 and 290 grams of carbs per day.

Protein: Did you know that every cell in the body contains protein and that muscle is mostly protein? The body does not store protein, so we must get it through outside sources. Protein helps to build muscle and to help us feel fuller longer. The recommendation is that 10% to 35% percent of total daily calories come from protein. For an 1,800 calorie diet, this equals 45-160 grams of protein per day.

Sources of complete protein are lean meat, fish, poultry, eggs and dairy products; and incomplete proteins include plant sources such as beans, peas, nuts, seeds, and grains. If you're always on the go, opt for an easy protein fix such as 10 almonds, a boiled egg, a small Greek yogurt or a spoonful of peanut butter. Unhealthy would be fatty meals (NY strip steak).

<u>Fat</u>: We need a certain amount of healthy fat in our diet. According to <u>myplate.gov</u> and other reference sources describing the Mediterranean Diet, healthy fats are found in vegetable oils, fatty fish, avocado, and nuts. Using many different sources and recommendations, I recommend three servings a day of these fats, spread throughout the day. Fat is needed for the health of our cells and can help us feel satisfied and full, with less of a tendency to reach for the simple carbohydrates and fill up on junk.

<u>Her is an example of a typical meal plan for me</u>: In the morning I have either brown rice crisp cereal with my homemade granola and almond milk, or a smoothie made with almond milk, almonds, frozen berries and frozen bananas. Mid-morning, I have either a protein bar or 10 almonds and an apple or banana.

For lunch I like a salad with spinach and arugula, a splash of olive oil and sprinkle of salt; vegetarian chicken nuggets, or leftover grilled chicken or fish from the night before; and whatever fresh veggies I have in the kitchen, mixed with a cup of brown rice or one-half of a sweet potato. For a mid-afternoon snack, I like some cold fresh veggies, like green beans or snap peas, some cocoa-dusted almonds, a big glass of water, and hot tea.

Dinner consists of a protein, salad, and hot vegetable (no starchy carbs), and later in the evening a cup of tea. This is my plan for most days.

On Fridays, I like a glass of wine or beer with dinner or popcorn at the movies. Saturdays might include dinner out with a starch, wine, or dessert, but not all three. On Sundays, I return back to the plan.

5. Fiber

Depending upon your age, you need 21-25 grams of fiber per day. According to the National Academy of Sciences, women under 50 should aim for 21 grams per day, while those over 50 need a bit more.

What is fiber? It's a substance in plant foods that the body cannot digest or absorb. Therefore, it passes virtually unchanged through the stomach and small intestine, and into the colon. People with diets high in fiber have a lower risk of diabetes, heart disease, or diverticulosis, constipation and colon cancer. Eating fiber-rich foods also helps you feel fuller longer after every meal, which can help curb overeating and weight gain.

There are two types of fiber:

Insoluble fiber promotes the movement of food through your digestive system and increases stool bulk, so it can be a benefit to those who struggle with constipation. Whole wheat flour, wheat bran, nuts and vegetables are good sources. It can be hard to get enough, and therefore, it is fine to take a supplement. Insoluble fiber is important in maintaining healthy bowel movements (BM). I talk to my patients frequently about bowel movements, and encourage healthy amounts of insoluble fiber as well as probiotics to maintain formed bowel movements.

An aspect of this which is not talked about enough is the link to vaginal health. Many women suffer from pain with intercourse and chronic vaginal discharge with bad odor and staining of the underwear. It is often from a bacteria imbalance and accidental BM soiling. It is not as if there are obvious pieces of BM in the vagina, but even an invisible, small amount of bacteria in the vagina can cause symptoms, especially if your estrogen is low and your vagina pH is higher than normal. Semen has a high pH, and if you have a little extra bad bacteria in your vagina, and you have intercourse without a condom, the higher pH makes the bad bacteria grow.

So it is important to keep your stools formed, rinse well with water after a loose stool, and see a health care provider if you have persistent stinky discharge. You may need a vaginal antibiotic to decrease the bad bacteria and allow for restoration of a healthy balance.

Soluble fiber, which dissolves in water, can help lower blood cholesterol and glucose levels, thus lowering the risk for cardiovascular disease and diabetes. You can get generous amounts of this in oats, peas, beans, apples, citrus fruits, carrots, rice, beans, barley and psyllium. Refined or processed foods are lower in fiber.

6. Activity—go the distance (10,000 steps per day for weight loss, aerobic fitness, and muscle building)

Activity is a big part of weight control, and it is time to examine your personal amount and type of activity. We need 5,000 steps a day to even think about maintaining our weight, and 10,000 steps per day to start to see weight loss. To maintain our metabolism, we must maintain or gain muscle, and there are a variety of programs to help you. For an overview, I recommend the book, Body for Life for Women: A Woman's Plan for Physical and Mental Transformation by Dr. Pamela Peeke. To maintain an activity, Dr. Peeke points out that it is important to like the activity. This seems really simple, but I see so many women try to force themselves, for example, to jog even if they hate to jog. It does not work!

Here's the good news: Even the smallest changes in your activity level can make a big difference. How do small bouts of exercise add up, and what kind of results can you expect to see in the grand scheme of things? By walking 10 minutes a day at a brisk pace, the average person (150 pounds) can expect to burn 60 calories. Repeating this activity everyday for a month would burn a total of 1,800 calories, or the number of calories required to burn off 0.5 lbs. of fat. Over the course of a year, this would result in a six-pound weight loss. Add to that healthful dietary changes and the possibilities increase exponentially.

Perimenopause can be the best wake-up call and the last opportunity to get it together. Once menopause sets in, there is a significant shift in the metabolism, and for many, it becomes very difficult to make changes. While it's never too late and never impossible to make changes, why wait until the effort required increases significantly? It is never too late! And don't forget the enervating effects of stress and sleep deprivation. If your body is in survival mode, how can you expect it to release weight? How can you expect the appetite signals to work right and have the energy for good food choices and workouts? All these aspects fit together like a puzzle, and knowledge gives you the power to see the big picture.

For myself, I have learned that I need an activity at least several times per week where I have to go all out—like running or swimming. If not, I am cranky and do not feel satisfied in my workout. But, I also need at least one session of yoga per week, and my favorite is Baron Baptiste. I own several DVDs and do it early in the morning before my kids can make fun of my bottom being in the air. If your budget allows, consider hiring a trainer, even for a few sessions, to teach you proper form and to aid in motivation.

7. Mind/Body—daily affirmation, gratitude and awareness of being present in your body

If you're feeling anxious, unmotivated, irritable, unable to focus, unhappy or uncharacteristically pessimistic, it's time to focus even more on your emotional and spiritual wellness. There are so many ways to fortify your spirit and all you have to do is find several emotionally satisfying strategies that work for you. I find it very helpful to keep a gratitude journal and recommend my patients do the same. Every day, can you write down what you are grateful for that day? Have three Go-To-Gratitudes, meaning you have three tear-jerking things you are grateful for (specific events that have happened) and you can remember those when you need them. You can change them if they start to lose their effectiveness.

Meditation, metered breathing, yoga and other exercises that relax, reenergize and revive your spirit and renew your optimism, are almost as important as sleep in reviving your body and mind. Sometimes a ten minute back rub at a salon is a quick antistress fix. Or, light a candle and sit quietly, take a walk in the woods or visit a museum. Do something that takes you away, even for 15 minutes, from your worries and stresses.

These SEEDS™ seem like common sense, but how many do we do every day? I do not even like to prescribe hormones or medication to treat PMS or depression without first prescribing a course of SEEDS™ alone. Medications can help modify or improve your system, but only with the other basics being supplied as well. Think of all the SEEDS™ as gas in the engine—without gas, the car cannot go, even if the engine is extra fancy, the tires brand new, or the paint is really shiny.

I see many women in the menopause clinic who are on hormone prescriptions and still have hot flashes. Or, they are unable to take hormones because they have had breast cancer or have risk factors, like heart disease or untreated high blood pressure. I do not increase their hormone dose or give hormones to those in whom it would not be safe, but instead help them think about how and where in their day to incorporate SEEDS™. Often, it just takes planning. When to drink the water (for teachers, nurses, or doctors) and when to empty their bladders. When to exercise, what menu to plan, and when to take vitamins and fiber. How to incorporate metered breathing and mindfulness. The plan will be different depending on circumstances. What amazes me is time after time, either communicated at the next office visit, or by a phone message or thank you note, the SEEDS™ work!

Chapter Seven

Tracking My Symptoms with the Menopause Transition Scale (MTS)

> "What would your life be like if you learned how to respect
> your body as though it were a precious creation
> —as valuable as a beloved friend?"
>
> ~Christiane Northrup, MD

It can happen to even the most well-intentioned midlife health reinventors. Work obligations derailed your early morning walk or run. Hot flashes kept you up all night and you were too tired to get on the treadmill in the morning. Your 13-year-old needed extra homework help before school and therefore your workout didn't happen. The phone rang and you raced to the ER to be with your mom. Before you knew it, your determination to eat right, exercise and get in a regular health routine was a distant memory.

Don't despair. We all get temporarily derailed now and then. The key is to kick-start your willpower and redirect yourself toward the healthy future you deserve. By using your dreams and goals as motivation, you can make good choices one day at a time. And you'll feel like a million bucks while you do it. As you develop healthier habits and implement small consistent changes, you'll feel more positive while feeling better, and your end result will be a long life with good health.

From my experience, and from the latest research, the women who fare the best during menopause with the fewest symptoms are the ones who are making good choices—doing their SEEDS™ and keeping their weight in the healthy range. By tracking your symptoms you can easily see what is making you feel good and what is not working.

Midlife, perimenopause and early menopause make up the perfect storm. As we move into planning our Life Action Plan (how we are going to put everything together to meet our goals), you will see that you actually have a choice in how you age, how long you live, and the quality of life you experience. Of course there are aspects we have no control over, but there are many aspects we do control. Hot flashes, night sweats and sleep disturbance are the gifts which tell us to get our act together.

Midlife/Menopause Transition Scale (MTS)

I've created a symptom scale, or Menopause Transition Scale (MTS), to help us keep track of midlife changes. Once you have completed the scale quiz (see page 120), you will have a measure of how you are faring. As you figure out a score, it is also a good time to think back on your day and remember what happened. Did the hot flash occur after you had a brownie or while you were arguing with your teenage daughter? Did you forget to bring your water bottle, and inadequate water led to you being sluggish and fatigued? By tracking your symptoms and then relating back to your SEEDS™, you will become aware of the patterns and be able to avoid the symptom the next day.

The language of the MTS came from my patients, and was tested in patient focus groups and in the W*A*I* Pointes™ Pilot study. Further research and validation of the scale is underway. Here is how to use the scale:

Hot flashes/night sweats

Are your hot flashes happening all the time, or never, or somewhere in between? Do they take you by complete surprise or can you predict them to happen after a hot cup of coffee or during a workout? Do you only have night sweats the night before the day your period starts or do night sweats occur almost every night?

Libido

This is a complex subject. The MTS is a good summary and written in language most women recognize right away. By keeping track of your MTS in this category, it becomes easy to track and relate to your cycle, menopause, life events, or relationship issues. And remember, some women are okay with an MTS 1 or MTS 2. This is not a judgment system, just a tracking system.

Weight

A simple weight tracking system has to make sense for you. I have had patients who struggle to maintain an MTS 3, but then realize that for them the level of exercise required and the dietary changes are not realistic. Therefore they will change their goal to an MTS 2, and be as healthy as possible in other areas of wellness.

Energy

Many women in menopause complain of low energy. Do you wake up refreshed and ready to go or do you hit the snooze buttons numerous times? Do you notice energy slumps during the day or do you generally feel energetic all day?

Moods

In this category, we are looking for whether your mood is bothering you, and how functional you feel in your environment. Are you a little down or anxious? Are you able to function and no one else is the wiser? Does your mood affect your motivation, your level of performance, and others close to you notice something is off? Understanding these aspects of your mood is the goal of this MTS scale.

Vaginal dryness/bladder complaints

Changes in your vaginal/vulvar/bladder health can have many causes, and are related to your anatomy, childbirth, hormones, bowel movements, activity level, physical fitness and exercise, and diet. In this MTS scale, we are looking for basic levels of function/dysfunction, and whether problems happen in a predictable way, i.e. with your cycle or menopause. Low estrogen can increase your chances of vaginal dryness and pain with intercourse, as well as bladder urgency and increased frequency of bladder infections. Stress incontinence or loss of urine with activity, laughing or sneezing is more of an anatomy issue, and happens more for women with a certain shaped pelvis who pushed a long time during childbirth. There are options for each condition, including the power of understanding what is going on and what is triggering the symptoms.

Vaginal Bleeding

A light regular bleeding cycle is like a vital sign for the body; it signals that everything is in good working order including hormones, nutrition, stress level, body weight, insulin levels, etc. An MTS 3 means that the bleeding pattern is normal, not bothersome, and predictable, as in light regular periods or menopause with no bleeding. An MTS 2 is predictable irregular periods such as occurs with perimenopause, or heavier, or more painful than normal bleeding.

However, it is not excessively interfering with life such as mandating missing work or daily activities, or losing excessive blood to cause anemia, etc. An MTS 1 indicates excessively heavy bleeding causing fatigue and excessive soiling of the clothes/car/bed. It is meeting the danger level in amount of flow such as having to change more than three products (pad or tampon) in one hour, number of days of bleeding (more than eight) or frequency (less than 14 days in between), bleeding after 12 months of no bleeding. An MTS 1 mandates evaluation by a gynecologist to confirm the cause is not cancer or pre-cancer, and to diagnose and treat the abnormality. Surgery is not always needed, as there are many options which do not involve surgery.

I have often seen women dealing with being an MTS 1, which is heavy, irregular bleeding resulting in embarrassing and distressing events of bleeding through clothes, bed sheets, and in the car—sometimes accepting excessively heavy bleeding as normal. They often have to call in sick to work, and it limits intimacy with their partner. Being an MTS 3 is great—either the bleeding is cyclical, predictable, and light. Or there is zero bleeding, as in after a hysterectomy, in menopause, or when using such products as the oral contraceptive pill, the progesterone-containing intrauterine device (IUD), or after an ablation. An MTS 2 means you might want to figure out and deal with the heavier bleeding, but it is not an emergency. I tell my patients that I can get bossy if I am concerned they have pre-cancer or cancer in their uterus; if they have anemia (low blood count), which is not safe or leading to fatigue and weakness; or if the symptoms are not conducive to a healthy lifestyle of exercise and good choices. They need to be bossy in terms of what they can live with in order to instigate an intervention with one of the tools-- medication or surgery.

Take the quiz to find out more about yourself! Circle which applies to you in each category and add up your score.

Dr. Diana L. Bitner, MD, NCMP

Scale Quiz

Hot flashes/night sweats

(3)--rare, predictable
(2)--moderate, predictable
(1)--frequent, unpredictable

Libido

(3)--both partners initiate, connected, playful
(2)--only partner initiation, relationship o.k.
(1) – rare, strained

Weight

(3) – stable, healthy or overweight, losing
(2) – overweight, not losing
(1) – obese or gaining

Energy

(3) – good, a.m. rested
(2) – mostly rested, good and bad days
(1) – mostly tired, poor function

Moods

(3) – good, minor cyclical or variations, predictable
(2) – cyclical, others notice, some dysfunction
(1) – mostly depressed or anxious, poor function

Vaginal Dryness/bladder complaints

(3) – minor dry, rare urgency
(2)--cyclical dryness, some leaking, urgency

(1) – dyspareunia (pain with sex), urgency

Vaginal Bleeding

(3) – cyclical, light
(2) – mod-heavy, predictable, mild pain
(1) – heavy, interfering, unpredictable, significant pain

Total
Score_____/21

Break it down

So how do you navigate midlife and menopause? First, track your symptoms by filling out an MTS score sheet every night before bed to record how the day went. If your score is not where you want, the first step is to go back to the SEEDS™ and think about what did not happen today.

What SEEDS™ did you not do—not enough water, not enough fiber, or inadequate exercise? Is it time to call your gynecologist to address bleeding or vaginal dryness or bladder leaking, or a Certified Menopause Practitioner to address menopause symptoms or decreased libido? In this day and age, we have many options to deal with such problems, and there is no reason to suffer. Midlife and early menopause is the time to get your act together. Being limited by heavy bleeding or debilitating hot flashes is not helpful to a long and happy life.

Dr. Diana L. Bitner, MD, NCMP

How to help your health care provider

Your MTS information can be very helpful for you in your annual physical with your physician. Or, it might lead you to find a physician, nurse practitioner, or midwife who is comfortable in helping you with symptoms of midlife or menopause. The website <u>menopause.org</u> offers a list of Certified Menopause Practitioners in your area, who often take common insurance and are looking to build their practice by taking care of women just like you!

This MTS tool can be the best use of time in such an office visit. For some women, by the time they see someone about their concerns, they have so many questions they don't know where to start!

For the doctor's part, it can help focus our efforts on a specific group of symptoms. Our first job is to make sure we are not missing another ailment such as thyroid dysfunction, diabetes, adrenal issues, etc. On your side, it helps you make sure your most pressing concerns are answered at that first visit and gives you a plan for future visits. You can start with the 1s and 2s, leaving the 3s for another time. Also, as you improve your SEEDS™ or add a prescription of hormones or serotonin, you can measure how you start to feel better!

Dr. Bitner's MTS Score:

Hot flashes/night sweats: No matter what I do, I am going to have the occasional symptom. I do not mind the occasional hot flash, which reminds me that I had too much sugar or forgot to keep up on my water during a busy day, but I do not want hot flashes embarrassing me during a patient visit or when I give a talk. I am okay with a rare or predictable hot flash or night sweat, as it can be a nice reminder of healthy habits. So, I want to be an MTS 3.

Libido: I like my husband and want this to be okay. So, I would prefer to be an MTS 3, and if not, I can ask why and work it out. Going back to the libido puzzle, I can look to figure out what piece is missing.

Weight: I definitely want to be an MTS 3. I am cranky and mad if I am not. So, either stable healthy or losing if I gained a bit over holidays or a vacation. That is my goal.

Energy: I want to be an MTS 3. That is, when the alarm goes off, I do not like the feeling of "ugh, I cannot bear to think about all I have to do today." I want to be ready to go—either to get on the spin bike downstairs or get in the shower before work.

Moods: I do not like myself when I am irritable, and act and feel as though no one can do anything right. I like the feeling that I can stick up for myself, and am able to say, "What about me?" instead of just taking care of everyone else, but I do not want to have the mean edge, which can happen when I am sleep deprived or feeling totally overwhelmed. I do not want to have to cope with more serious anxiety and depression; these conditions can severely limit women's ability to function and be successful—for themselves and those people around them. An MTS 3 means I feel good on the inside as well as out. An MTS 2 means I am functional and okay to the public, but not great on the inside or to my private/safe people. An MTS 1 means it is bad for all involved.

Vaginal Dryness: I have seen many women have an MTS 1 in this category. I do not want that for my patients or myself! I want to be an MTS 3. This means no pain with intercourse, rare and predictable leaking only; for example, if I have had too much coffee and got laughing before I could make it to the bathroom. I want to be able to exercise, laugh, and sneeze without urine running down my leg, and without frequent bladder or vaginal infections.

Dr. Diana L. Bitner, MD, NCMP

Vaginal bleeding: I don't have to have irregular, heavy periods, so I have taken steps to not have any periods. I have chosen an option to avoid having heavy, irregular periods.

Chapter Eight

Treating Symptoms with Modern Knowledge

"Midlife is an exciting opportunity to surrender to your true self."

~Joan Borysenko

Dear Dr. Diana Bitner,

I wanted to send a quick note to first thank you for your time and recommendations from my appointment with you on June 11. I was so impressed with your knowledge and passion for women's health, especially in regards to menopause. I thank you for the generous amount of time you spent with me and for what you taught me!

I have incorporated the 7 SEEDS into my routine and am now getting 7 hours of sleep a night, eating less sugar, eating more dietary fiber, and drinking a lot more water (but I don't think I am quite up to 80 ounces yet). I continue to exercise and have my quiet time every morning. I feel great overall, my hot flashes are now minimal and my vaginal dryness much improved!

With regards to the medications you recommended:

1. I completed the 6 days of metronidazole vaginal gel for the bacteria infection
2. Now that I am putting the Estrace cream inside the vagina, I am not having the itchy reaction. I never started the other estrogen-type cream your nurse called in from about a week ago.
3. I am applying the Vivelle dot patch every 3 days.
4. I am taking the progesterone 100 mg pill once a day, which I do think helps my sleep quality.
5. I started the Fibercon 1 tablet/day.

We discussed starting Lexapro, an antidepressant, for 3 months to increase my serotonin levels. I decided not to start this because I feel good and don't want any of the potential side effects from Lexapro. I did fill the script but then never started on the medication. I thought you might want this info for my medical record.

I look forward to my follow up visit with you in a few months. I will be curious on what your assessment is from the pathology report from my polyp that was removed during my ablation in 2003.

I hope you have a fabulous summer! Thank you again for helping me feel my best! May God continue to bless your work.

Sincerely,

(Actual patient of Dr. Bitner, used with permission)

Modern medicine

I do not know if I could have been a physician in the era before antibiotics, ultrasound machines, safe surgery, and cancer-fighting chemotherapy—it would have been so hard to feel helpless in the face of suffering and disease.

As a traditionally-trained physician from Wayne State University, I like to start with minimal intervention and ramp up a treatment plan as necessary. I strive to apply knowledge from all cultures and medicine practices, including the shiny halls of NIH-funded research labs. I see MRI machines, surgery and medicines as tools at my disposal—gifts which allow for the treatment and prevention of disease. Of course, while I would rather help patients prevent a heart attack or diabetes with only a balanced diet and exercise, there are many situations when medicine and surgery are necessary. In this day and age, realism is necessary.

I have delivered thousands of babies in the hospital setting and am so glad to be a physician in this day and age. We try to keep the environment as calm, natural, and non-medical as possible. As a result, I have seen many babies come into this world in a home-like and calm setting, with only myself, the delivery nurse, and the parents present. At the same time, I was confident in the fact that there was modern technology, an operating room, and a team of capable and well-qualified nurses and doctors behind the wall, as well as a world-class neonatal nursery just down the hall. In the instances when the baby's heart tones slowed to dangerous levels or there were other complications, I could intervene and save a baby who otherwise could have died from abruption or uterine rupture. Modern medicine brings security and treatment options to my practice.

Preventable illness increases during perimenopause and early menopause. It is a time when the internal landscape is changing again, similar to both puberty and pregnancy. Hormones, body chemistry and lifestyle habits meet together in the perfect storm. Many women emerge from the storm well, others not so well. The result depends on how healthy she was when the storm started, how she was able to cope with the storm elements, and the history of women in her family who went before.

Let us think about an average American woman I might see in my office. She went to college or started work out of high school. Maybe she got married and had babies, or got involved in work and community. Either way, she was very busy in her 20s and 30s and her health took a back seat while she gave to others instead of herself. Then came the 40th birthday, and her weight became harder to lose, and midlife symptoms started—sleep disturbances, heavy periods, mood changes, etc. Some of her symptoms were from aging, some were from hormone changes, but most were rooted in her lifestyle habits of being over-scheduled, over-tired and overweight.

When I see a patient who fits this description, my first goal is to empower her with the knowledge of what a healthy lifestyle can do to cure much of what ails her. We would look at which barriers prevent success. Perhaps it is her heavy periods. There are times when the situation requires at least short term tools, such as surgery for heavy bleeding, or SSRI medications to get brain chemicals up to functional levels, or short-term hormone replacement to treat the night sweats and allow for adequate sleep and therefore an early morning workout. Another barrier could be that she is genetically geared towards obesity and diabetes. If a woman who had gestational diabetes is now fighting central obesity, sugar cravings, and facial hair, and is too far down the road of prediabetes to where only a medication like Metformin will help with the insulin resistance, so be it. I would rather prescribe a medication—after considering the pros and cons—that would allow her to turn back the clock before diabetes sets in and is too late to prevent her heart attack.

Therefore, there are many times when I believe it is appropriate to consider the risks and benefits of prescription treatment. I employ evidence-based medicine in my practice and feel strongly about "safety first." Any prescription comes with a discussion about the risks and benefits, expected outcomes, and a followup appointment.

Treatment Options for Perimenopause and Menopause

- Lifestyle
- Birth control pill
- Estrogen pills, patches, and gels
- Progesterone pills, patches, and intrauterine devices (IUD)
- Non-FDA approved testosterone cream
- Serotonin Medications
- Herbal Remedies
- Avoidance of symptom triggers

Who cannot take hormones? Women who have:

- Breast cancer
- High risk for heart disease or stroke
- Heart disease or prior stroke

- High risk for blood clot in legs or lungs
- Past history of blood clot in legs or lungs
- More than 10 years have passed since last menstrual period
- Unexplained vaginal bleeding

Hormone Basics

A key hormone in women's well-being is estrogen which is made in the ovary and to a lesser extent in belly fat. Estradiol is the principle form of estrogen made and is the most potent estrogen in our body; the other two forms are estriol and estrone. Estrogen can only work in body tissues that have estrogen receptors. When estrogen binds to a receptor, the receptor gets activated and starts a chain reaction in the cell which contained the receptor. The specific action that occurs is determined by what cell and area of the body tissue we are talking about, as well as the woman's age and ovarian aging status.

There are estrogen receptors almost everywhere—in the uterus, skin, bones, breast, fat, and brain. For example, when the estrogen receptor is activated in the uterus, the uterus lining is stimulated to grow. In the breast, glandular cells are made to proliferate and develop. In the brain, chemical levels such as serotonin are regulated, and in the ovary, regulation with feedback occurs. Estrogen and progesterone are both hormones made by the ovaries and each has many actions all over the body.

For example, think of the inside of your uterus as a lawn. Estrogen acts as a fertilizer, and progesterone acts as the weed killer. Abnormal bleeding happens when the lawn is too long, too short, or very uneven, which occurs with too much estrogen, not enough progesterone, or uneven levels of both. In menopause, the lining of the uterus should be as short and even as a putting green--without crabgrass or weeds (polyps or cancer). In other conditions such as PCOS (polycystic ovarian syndrome), which is marked by consistently high estrogen levels and low progesterone levels, the lining of the uterus is like a lawn that has not been mowed for months, thick and gone to seed. Uterine precancer is synonymous to crab grass, and uterine cancer is crabgrass which has spread to the sidewalk.

Another key hormone is testosterone. Testosterone is made in the ovary, the adrenal gland, and from estrogen stored in belly fat. Testosterone in healthy levels can contribute to motivation for life and sex drive. Too much testosterone, which can result from conditions such as PCOS or excess belly fat, can lead to facial hair, anger outbursts and high cholesterol.

When hormone levels are normal, most of us do not even stop to think about our hormone levels. We take them for granted, and do not even consider all that is happening because of their presence. Because of hormones, women are able to feel and function as expected. But hormones also contribute to mood, metabolism, sleep patterns, sex drive, bone health, healthy vaginal skin, bladder function, bleeding patterns, ability to become pregnant, etc.

Estrogen, progesterone and testosterone also affect our physiology. For example, when our levels drop, as in menopause, our heart disease risk starts to match that of men. Women who take too much testosterone in menopause not only can have crazy aggression issues and hair growth, but also high levels of cholesterol. Estrogen can help our ability to handle sugar and appetite for sugar, as well as keep our tissue healthy and elastic, such as in the blood vessel walls around our heart. When our hormone levels fall below the levels to which we are accustomed, all of these same functions are changed. When the hormone levels are low, up to 80% of women experience symptoms and some distress from symptoms like fatigue, mood change, or altered sleep patterns; 20% do not have many symptoms at all.

The women I see who are least affected by menopause symptoms are those who are living a healthy lifestyle: their weight is healthy, they are very active and exercise regularly, eat a diet low in sugar or simple carbohydrates, drink minimal alcohol and plenty of water, and have little stress. The more stress and bad habits, the more likely they are to have hot flashes.

Women of certain ethnicity and socioeconomic background tend to experience the symptoms very differently from others. A large study called the SWAN Study was done to better understand how a variety of women experience menopause. For example, women of Asian descent were found to not complain of or talk about hot flashes, but instead had issues with mood changes and depression. Caucasian and African American women tend to have more hot flashes.

Again, perimenopause and menopause are the perfect storms. When hormone-related changes occur in our body, symptoms such as sugar cravings meet up with hormone-related symptoms such as night sweats, and poor sleep, weight gain and diabetes can be the result. I am talking about midlife-perimenopause weight gain, development of early diabetes, increasing plaque in heart blood vessels leading to an increased risk for a heart attack, and low hormones leading to low brain chemicals and therefore poorer coping skills and depression or anxiety. It is a merry-go-round that can be hard to get off.

For example, we know that if a woman has her ovaries out before the age of 45 and does not take estrogen, her risk of a heart attack or stroke is much higher than if she had taken estrogen, and therefore, the development of heart disease will happen earlier than if her ovaries had been left in place. What happens in midlife during the transition into menopause will determine how the rest of life will go. At menopause, for most women, their health is as good as it will get. That is why we need to act in midlife.

All women who are in perimenopause or early menopause could benefit from an appointment with a Certified Menopause Practitioner (menopause.org). It is an opportunity to use the symptoms as a signal that the body is changing, and not all for the better. It is a time to look at lifestyle habits (SEEDS™ see Chapter Six), catalog the symptoms, and untangle the web of what is causing what.

What about Using Hormones?

If the symptoms interfere with your day or your sleep to the point of leaving you distracted, experiencing poor concentration or having increased depressive or anxious feelings, hormone supplementation in very low doses can be effective.

There are rules about safe dosing so you should consult your health care provider to help determine what the best dosage is for you. The goal is to use the lowest possible dose, the baseline amount we need to feel like ourselves. Be very aware that your hormone levels may fluctuate and you and your health care provider should be prepared to be flexible.

For some, estrogen at the lowest effective dose could be the best decision. A treatment plan should include specific expected outcomes, how long the hormone should be taken, and a plan for healthy lifestyle.

The best treatment is to step back, understand what's going on and return to the basics of self-care.

Hormone Medications

The intention here is to discuss the use of prescription therapies for menopause symptoms and appropriate expectations of their use. This information is meant to be a primer on the treatment options for midlife and menopause symptoms, not a guide for you to self-treat. For additional information on what options are best for you, I recommend going to the website for the North American Menopause Society (menopause.org) and investigate for yourself, as well as finding a Certified Menopause Provider in your area. The information on the website is as free from bias as possible and very well-rounded.

Estrogen

Estrogen can be given in different forms, including oral pills, patches, spray, and cream. When it is taken in forms that cross the skin, there is the least effect on the liver and reduces the more serious risks of blood clots and stroke. Estrogen you take could be identical to your natural estrogen or isolated from horse urine or plant products. The products recommended by the North American Menopause Society are FDA-approved hormone products with controlled dosing. What that means is when I prescribe a given pill or patch, I have peace of mind you will receive a pure product in the amount described on the label.

The term bioidentical can be confusing. To health care providers and chemists, bioidentical means the medicine prescribed contains hormones which are identical to the estradiol and progesterone made by the ovary. Such hormone medications are available in FDA-approved, metered dosing products covered by insurance. But, too often, non-FDA approved medicines are marketed under the label bioidentical to falsely imply the product has a better safety record.

If you take estrogen, and you have a uterus (have not had a hysterectomy), then you need to take progesterone as well. History has taught us that estrogen alone can cause uterine cancer. And, studies show that women who take hormone replacement therapy (HRT) with progesterone have a lower risk of uterine cancer than women who do not take HRT at all. We know from research how much progesterone is needed to keep the uterus safe and studies that look at compounded progesterone cream prove there is not uterine cancer prevention.

Dr. Diana L. Bitner, MD, NCMP

Hormone Replacement Therapy (HRT)

With hormone replacement therapy, the goal is to reduce symptoms without increasing the risk of complications. The key word is replacement, meaning not to triple the levels of estrogen your ovary used to make. Our goal is to use the lowest dose for the least amount of time necessary to treat the worst symptoms, and to start the therapy early in the menopause transition. To determine the correct dose for you, we only need to know your phase of ovarian function and your symptoms. Blood levels are rarely needed to determine a plan.

The safety of taking hormones has been questioned over the years. When hormones were first given in the 1960s, it was not understood that progesterone was needed to be given with estrogen in order to avoid uterine cancer. Four percent of women who had a uterus and did not take progesterone developed uterine cancer; the practice of prescribing hormones was therefore stopped. After safe dosing was determined to prevent uterine cancer, the practice of prescribing hormones was resumed. Then, in 1993, the WHI Study was published and the media hyped the data that more women who took estrogen over those who did not developed more breast cancer. The number of prescriptions for HRT dropped dramatically all over the world, and many women suffered as a consequence.

Women who were on estrogen alone (they had no uterus) did not get more breast cancer. And the women who did get more breast cancer were over 65, on both estrogen and synthetic progesterone, and had not taken hormones for years after menopause until they started it for the study. Also, the number of women who got more breast cancer was small—four more per 10,000 women. That certainly wasn't trivial if you were one of the four, but also should not keep the thousands of women who would benefit from taking hormones.

The WHI Study was begun by Dr. Jacques Rossoux. He is a researcher from South Africa who was interested in heart disease, specifically in the practice of whether hormones should be given to women after menopause to reduce the risk of heart attack. At the time the study was begun, many doctors gave hormones with that expectation. The study showed that hormones actually increased the risk of a heart attack in women who had not been on hormones for over 10 years before starting, who had metabolic syndrome (obesity, high blood pressure, high cholesterol and high blood sugar), or had significant pre-existing risks for heart attack. On the other hand, the risk of heart disease was lowered for women who started the hormones soon after menopause and had low risk for heart disease or stroke.

What has come out of all of this information is the timing hypothesis. It means that if you are going to take hormones, then you should start in perimenopause or menopause and stay healthy. I tell my patients, "If you want to keep getting your hormones, keep the weight off, keep your blood pressure down, and stay off the sugar." Such advice is usually a good motivator.

What can you expect from taking hormone replacement therapy? It is FDA-approved for reduction of hot flashes, night sweats, to protect your bones form thinning, or osteoporosis, and to avoid vaginal dryness and pain with intercourse. It is used off-label for improving libido, mild to moderate mood disturbance (not severe depression or anxiety), and aiding with sleep. Estrogen is NOT a weight loss drug and should not be expected to help you lose weight. Estrogen can help with sleep which can help with the motivation to exercise and therefore lose weight, but it does not directly cause weight loss.

Birth Control Pill

The birth control pill contains estrogen and progesterone at three times the level found in hormone replacement therapy, but still in safe levels for women in perimenopause who do not smoke. For many women, the birth control pill is a great way to deal with the symptoms of perimenopause, such as mood swings, heavy irregular bleeding, and menstrual migraine headaches, as well as provide birth control. There are also healthy side effects to taking birth control, such as lowering the risk of ovarian cancer and bad cholesterol levels. The downside of the birth control pill is that oral estrogen can reduce mid-cycle sex drive by binding up free testosterone in the blood.

Again, for more information, find a Certified Menopause Practitioner in your area and check out the website menopause.org.

Non-hormone therapy: SSRIs/SNRIs

Non-hormone therapy such as Selective Serotonin and Serotonin-norepinephrine Reuptake Inhibitors (SSRIs) has been traditionally prescribed for depression and anxiety. These medicines work by increasing the levels of natural brain chemicals that can be decreased with unresolved stress, inadequate sleep, and lower than normal estrogen levels. Hot flashes often improve quickly for many women who take these medications and can be a welcome relief for women who cannot, or wish not, to take hormone medication. Side effects of SSRIs/SNRIs include agitation in a small percentage of women that tends to go away with time; at high doses these meds can slow the heart rate and cause dizziness and fainting. For some women, these meds reduce sex drive and makes orgasm more difficult. Some of the medicines in this class are more effective than others and also have fewer side effects; consult a Certified Menopause Practitioner for the best choice for you. When these medications are prescribed for PMS mood symptoms, mild depression or mild anxiety, the effects can take longer to notice than for hot flashes.

Gabapentin is an old, but strong, drug used for nerve pain and to prevent seizures. It can be very effective for hot flashes in some women, especially those who tolerate the sedating side effects. Usually the symptoms of dizziness and sedation resolve after a week or two of therapy, and can be an option.

Non-prescription Therapies

Non-prescription therapies have not been proven to be as effective as prescription therapies, but are likely to be safe. For example, Vitamin B deficiencies are rare, but taking a Vitamin B complex is safe, and some women swear by it for hot flashes. Vitamin D deficiency can cause osteoporosis and studies are ongoing to understand what doses are best, depending on where you live and your body fat percentage. Some women would claim that it helps with symptoms of fatigue, aches and pains. Again, a generally accepted dosage is 2,000 IU per day; no harm is likely and there is great potential benefit.

The best way to get vitamins is to eat a balanced diet with at least five servings of vegetables and fruit per day, including dairy products and leafy greens to provide calcium, as well as eggs and meat to provide Vitamin B. Fish oil from fatty fish such as salmon, sardines, and black cod has been shown to lower triglycerides, a form of fat which circulates in the blood and increases risk for heart disease.

Non-prescription, over-the-counter hormones such as progesterone cream, come in very different doses and forms, and have mixed effects. Such creams do not protect the uterus when taking estrogen for hot flashes, but have not been shown to cause harm otherwise. We do not know whether they can hurt someone with a progesterone-dependent breast cancer; however, I would not recommend taking the chance. Again, safety first.

DHEA is a pre-hormone for testosterone and similar hormones. In women, it is made mostly in the adrenal glands, but also in the ovaries. As the natural levels fall with age, some have proclaimed a strong anti-aging effect. However, studies have not shown good proof of this claim. Oral therapy needs to be metabolized by the liver, and patches and creams will give a more constant level. Taking DHEA has been shown helpful for sex drive in women with proven low levels of DHEA, but not in healthy counterparts. Currently, studies are being done with vaginal DHEA for women in menopause to improve the hormonal aspect of sex drive. DHEA has been shown to raise levels of testosterone as well as estrogen and estrone; therefore, it should not be used by women who have had breast cancer. Also, DHEA is not safe in childbearing-age women who could become pregnant, as it could make a female baby have male characteristics.

CAM: Complementary and Alternative Medicine

The most commonly used alternative therapy for hot flashes has been soy. It is an isoflavone-containing food, a class of plant chemicals which bind to estrogen receptors. Soy can turn the receptors on or off, depending on the tissue and receptor type. There are several different types of isoflavones found in soy preparations, and the relative amount of each can determine its effectiveness. And, not all of us can metabolize the isoflavones to equol (30% of North American women can) which is the actual compound that binds to the receptor. Only half of women not raised on a soy-based diet from birth can metabolize soy products in equol. Equol is the active compound that binds to the estrogen receptor and helps with hot flashes and other menopausal symptoms.

Soy has been shown to have only limited effect on lowering cholesterol, but more study trials are underway. Some studies show some benefit for reducing hot flashes, while others do not. When just equol was used, there was more positive effect; if you are someone who converts soy to equol, the reduction effect would be greater. There has been no positive effect on vaginal dryness, and no detrimental effect on the lining of the uterus or breast tissue.

Herbs such as Black Cohosh are in wide use for hot flash reduction as over-the-counter products under various names and brands. Such products are sold as dietary supplements and not monitored for purity or concentration. It is not known how Black Cohosh works, although it is the most widely studied herb for hot flash reduction. In only rare cases can it hurt your liver, and for some women, especially in very early menopause, it can be helpful for hot flashes. Large studies do not show a strong effect, but if taken, effects should be seen by one month of use.

St. John's Wort is an herb used for depression; it is not known for sure how it works, but thought to be related to serotonin medications. It has not been shown to be effective for severe depression, but positive for mild to moderate mood disturbance. Taking it with prescription serotonin medications could increase the risk of serotonin syndrome, a potentially dangerous condition of muscle twitching and seizure. It also can increase sun-sensitivity. However, at usual doses, it is unlikely to cause harm, and could be effective.

Valerian is an herb that has been shown to be helpful for insomnia; in Germany and by the WHO (World Health Organization), it is recognized for insomnia and nervousness. For best effect it should be taken at bedtime for more than several weeks and there are no serious side effects.

Chapter Nine

Creating My Life Action Plan

"Women now facing midlife are different than any other generation."

~Leon Speroff, MD

Getting It Together

I created W*A*I* Pointes™ (see Chapter Three) using a foundation of goal setting and built it up with exercises and assessments to help you plot where you are now, your Place in Process (PIP) and Picture of Self (POS). By combining these self-appraisals and snapshots, you are able to create your Life Action Plan. This is the personalized plan you'll stick with as you journey through midlife and menopause.

In my view, for a plan to work over time, it has to be specific to you, reward you with short term results, and show you a way to overcome barriers that keep you from living to your potential. A health plan has to be one that you design to fit your goals, your lifestyle, and your ability.

A successful program starts slowly and builds gradually. If we can break it down into categories, we can make the overall process manageable. Also, we can understand how actions in one area affect another. We see how small everyday choices affect our big picture and our best path.

The idea is simple: Set goals.

W*A*I*Pointes™ is based on each of us connecting with clear goals for our future. For some, this is easy. But for others, goals have gotten lost in the day-to-day survival. Once we reestablish clear goals and think about how we want to live in the future, daily choices become more significant. It gives us a clear starting point—we see where we are and make a plan for the end game, our healthy future.

Creating Your Comeback Plan

I doubt if any of us graduate from high school saying, "I am going to gain 50 lbs., smoke a pack of cigarettes day, sit around, suffer from depression, or have a heart attack before 50." So how does that happen to many women?

It is often a gradual thing, a decline in habits and health, slowly adding up. So, today, no matter where you are on your Life Action Plan, we are here to get you back on your path. We are done with regret and self blame, so let us start fresh. First, what is your POS?

Second, your PIP will give you a freeze-frame view of where you are now and your position on the Life Action Plan. You can then decide if you are okay with where you are, now that you understand how being overweight, inactive, and overstressed can affect your future possibilities. And then, you can decide your future. What changes are you willing to make to have the life you want ten or twenty years from now? What will you do to achieve that quality of life? What is your Life Action Plan in terms of health success?

W*A*I* Pointes™ is not a plan I create for you. It is a plan you create for you, while I, through this book, serve as your guide. As a physician, I can diagnose and treat heart disease, obesity, hypertension, bleeding troubles and other disease, but I want to do more than hold your hand and write prescriptions. I want to give you the tools to live your life as fully and healthfully as possible.

This is about your plan for the future. I want you to say, "This is my plan," and consider the book as a way to help you go faster and farther toward your goals. We need to get attached to the future and connect with our future selves. Once we understand what it is that we want, and develop that picture, we then have a goal to work towards.

You Can Do It!

Let's start creating your Life Action Plan. This is a tool to chart your progress and create clear, visual goals and remind yourself of your path.

Make it Last: Create a Five-Step Plan

You've made it this far and have your goals lined up. Transform your goals into action and build the momentum by setting up a five-step plan:

- Dream it
- Research it
- Decide action plan
- Determine logistics
- Put it on the calendar to execute it

Journal each of these steps, asking yourself questions about what this will look like for you to achieve your goals. Start a daily journal to record your process and reassess your progress. What works? What doesn't work? What are your barriers and what steps do you take to overcome your barriers?

Dr. Diana L. Bitner, MD, NCMP

Here's How the Life Action Plan Works

Example: Heart Disease. You have determined your POS and done your PIP and other assessments. So, take H (heart disease). First, write out your PIP freehand: "I want to be active, able to hike the dunes with my kids; I do not want to be told, "You have heart vessel disease and you could have a heart attack;" I would worry about leaving my kids without their mom.

I want my cholesterol to be good: HDL >60, LDL <100, triglycerides ≥100, CRP 1.0, waist circumference ≥34 inches, BMI ≥ 25 and body fat percentage ≥ 25%. I want to be able to exercise more than 30 minutes without having to stop.

That is where the Life Action Plan comes in. It is a chart that compares the POS with the PIP in each category and also a line on that category for the personalized recommendation for that person based on what options the patient chooses.

Another example: Strong bones. So, let's say your POS for strong bones is to be a 3 = No risk factors that are in your control, good numbers on DEXA, a bone density scan (if applicable), and having a minimal fall risk. But, your PIP is a 2. You and your physician then look at your risk factors, and make a plan how you can reduce them. If your risk factor is smoking, will you choose to quit or reduce the number of cigarettes you smoke in a day? What is the plan to change your PIP of a 2 into your POS of 3?

Are you on thyroid medicine? Make sure your blood levels are in normal range. Not having enough physical activity? Then do 50 jumping jacks every day with your shoes off to keep your spine and hips strong. Forgetting to take your calcium and Vitamin D? "Make it easy to remember, not easy to forget" (see next page). Then, chart, recheck, and have your DEXA every two years and recalculate PIP every month. If the PIP and the POS do not match up, then make a plan to change.

"Make it hard to forget, not hard to remember," goes along with the concept of pokeoke. Pokeoke is a Japanese manufacturing term which means making the right thing to do the easy thing to do, or to mistake-proof a process. So, for example, I pokeoke the taking of my Vitamin D supplement. I put it in my makeup bag, next to my mascara, and take it before I make my coffee. How do I remember my thyroid medicine? It is next to my toothbrush. My calcium and Vitamin D are in the car so I take them in the morning and on the way home at night. The goal is to make it all hard to forget, not hard to remember.

One more example: Ease of Coping. We calculate your PIP, using several scores including a PHQ-9 and COPE Scale. For example, a POS in this category of 3 means you are able to cope when times get tough or you encounter challenges, you are able to keep a positive outlook, and have a group of friends who support each other and you call them should you need help.

If you do not have a 3 in the Coping category, how could you increase your score? There are proven ways to do this.

How to go from a 2 to a 3 Life Action Plan (LAP):

- Connect with positive friends.
- Practice positive thinking.
- Ask your doctor about PMS, and address if you have a family history of poor coping or history of postpartum depression.
- Be aware that there is a higher chance of PMS and perimenopause depression if you had postpartum depression.
- Be clear about what is on your mind when you wake up and can't sleep. Is it bills you cannot pay? Are you in a relationship that is abusive, or you are not treated as an equal? Is

there a relationship you have neglected? Are you bothered by dirty closets or clutter?
- Make time for yourself. For me, I accomplish two things at once: exercise is time for me to listen to my music and read my magazines; it is a great stress reliever that I even have energy for at 10:00 p.m. because I can put on the earphones and jam for even 10 minutes. Pampering does not have to be expensive or away from the family.

The key to filling out your Life Action Plan is to match it to what works in your life—and what you know won't work. Staying on track—and recording your process—is an important key to success.

What's Essential for You to Make This Happen?

When I started to notice how women were not connected to their future, it hit me. If I can get women to think about their future, maybe it will make a difference. I was right. In my office, I started asking my patients, "What did you dream of when you were 13, 18 or 22? What were your dreams when you graduated from high school? Has your life turned out like you wanted? In this land of opportunity, why have you not gotten everything you ever wanted?" As I have asked these questions more and more, I have learned that many of my patients have not thought of their dreams for years and almost feel reminiscent when calling up the memory.

Whether the future is short-term or long-term, such as in giving birth to a healthy baby, or as a woman reaching the age of 60 and feeling healthy, I want to make sure my patient and I have a plan.

My goal is to help you see what is hard for you, understand why, and get back on the path you hoped for. If you are on your path, let's talk about how to maintain your path with great vitality and health. I have learned that most women are alike. We do not want to be told what to do, or be given a prescription for pills and sent on our way. We want to know what we are up against and then we can deal with it. Some want more detail than others, but most want at least to be offered the explanation.

Now Get Started

It's high time we change our views about the 'change of life' and accept that it's a normal, natural event that all women experience if they are lucky to live into their forties and beyond. This is a medical fact; it's not a discussion. Menopause is not a disease any more than pregnancy is a disease. Yes, the bodily changes and side effects can be unpleasant, but need not be disabling. Menopause is not a synonym for memory lapses, mysterious symptoms, lack of sex drive, depression or the countless other symptoms attributed to this misunderstood phase.

Menopause is not nature's way of announcing that your life as a vital, sexy, sassy woman is over. To the contrary, I see menopause as nature's invitation to redefine your life, recapture your energy and redirect your course of life over 50. Still, if you are unsure if you should be jumping for joy when the PMS cramps and periods stop, or collapsing in tears because those monthly affirmations of youth and fertility are over, you are not alone.

More Willpower to You

What does owning our power mean? It means living true and being true to yourself. How do you know your purpose? It takes time and an open heart and mind, without resting on the labels other people put on us. It takes time to trust what feels right, and to slowly build on small realizations of being on the right path. It does not mean being perfect, it does not mean always being right, and it does not mean getting your way or being so powerful as to extend your will on others.

How do dreams and health goals come together? In midlife, we get a second chance to examine what we have done with our lives and decide what the future will hold. Whether you look back with regret or satisfaction, moving forward requires learning from the past and having a vision for your future. Common sense would tell us that having goals, such as meeting Mr. Right or getting a big promotion, are impossible to accomplish if you do not feel good. Women, who are fit and healthy and understand their changing bodies, are more apt and able to be in touch with their path. Think of women who make second careers or become successful in a career after their children are grown. They tend to have their health figured out. I think of Heidi Klum, Christine Northrop or Maria Shriver; these women have become successful after 40 and are obviously fit and healthy. Such health does not just happen; they work hard to look and feel good and can subsequently focus on their creative endeavors. I want to help you do the same.

You might not consciously have decided on an ideal body weight, cholesterol level or a desire to be cancer free, but you may see other women and think, *Why doesn't she look tired?* or *I wish I was thin like her.* Or if you see a woman with a kerchief covering her head as a result of chemo, you may think, Oh my God, I can't imagine. Reminders of what we want, or do not want, are all around. Success does not just happen on its own. Little bits of wishful thinking do not make great things happen. It is what comes after the wishful thinking that counts.

Start your new health life plan now. Map your dream, your goals and the challenges ahead, and get started.

Sample of a Life Action Plan

	POS	PIP	Risks Identified	Recommendations
Activity			Barriers: Time Fatigue Family resp. Dislike activity	• 150 min moderate activity/week (aerobic + strength) • 10,000 steps/day for wt loss • 5,000 steps/day for maintenance • Strength training 3+ times/week
Obesity			BMI≥30 Waist circumference ≥35" W:H ratio ≥0.85 Body fat %≥35%	• Achieve healthy weight • Consider food diary if not doing already • 5 srvs fruit/veggies/day • Keep track of SEEDS™
Cancer				
Lung			None	• 5 srvs fruit/veggies/day • Report symptoms to PCP *(changing cough, cough blood, chest pain, shortness of breath, unexplained weight loss)*
Colon			≥2 srvs red meat/week ≥7 alcoholic drinks/week Low level physical activity Family hx colon polyps	• ≤3 srvs red meat/week • Decrease alcohol intake • Moderate physical activity 3 hours/week (walking counts!) • Report symptoms to PCP *(rectal bleeding, new onset diarrhea/constipation, change in stool appearance, abdominal pain)*
Breast			BMI ≥30 ≥7 alcoholic drinks/week Low level physical activity	• Continue regular mammograms & monthly self breast exams • Report changes in lumps • Achieve healthy weight • Decrease alcohol intake • Moderate physical activity 3 hours/week (walking counts!)

Diabetes			BMI ≥30 Waist circumference ≥35" W:H ratio ≥0.85 Body fat% ≥35%	• Achieve healthy weight initially aim for loss of 5-10% of body wt • Avoid simple carbohydrates • Decrease alcohol intake • Annual fasting blood sugar • Increase physical activity
Ease of coping			Poor role model Depression	• Counseling • Problem solving • Consider medications as needed
Phase of ovarian function			Depression	• Continue effexor, report worsening symptoms to PCP
Good bones			Low level physical activity	• Calcium and vitamin D daily • Weight bearing activity at least 30 min 3x/wk • 50 jumps/day • Bone density screening when postmenopausal
Heart disease			HDL (good cholesterol) ≤50 Elevated CRP (inflammation) Triglycerides ≥150 Waist circumference ≥35" W:H ratio ≥0.85 ≥7 alcoholic drinks/week	• Achieve healthy weight • 150 min moderate activity/wk • Consider omega 3 fatty acid supplement (fish oil or flaxseed) • Decrease alcohol intake • Report any symptoms to PCP *(chest pain, shortness of breath, activity intolerance, unusual fatigue, other vague symptoms)*
Income security			No safety net	• Meet with financial planner • Build budget • Build safety net ≥6 mo expenses • Spend within means • Pay off credit card debt

Chapter Ten

Healthy Aging in an Unhealthy World

"There's 'intelligent aging' and then there's just 'getting older.'"

~Dr. Diana L. Bitner, MD, NCMP
Medical Director, Spectrum Health Medical Group
Midlife and Menopause Health Services

Healthy aging is about making choices to be as well as possible, and when things happen out of your control, the choices you have made help you meet them with resiliency.

You've made it this far in the book: figured out your Place in Process (PIP), developed your Picture of Self (POS), created your Life Action Plan, and now you're mulling the options for making it happen. When you think about the changes you want to make in your fitness and wellness routines, there are a myriad of excuses you can grab for. It's the same fight you've been having in your head for years. This means you are going to have to disrupt your routine, get rid of your excuses and start doing things differently.

The results can be extraordinary. You will look in the mirror one day at the person you envisioned you wanted to be in your POS. Now it is time to start small and be creative.

The Life Action Plan is designed to take the mystery out of midlife transition. Every woman is different from another because of her family history, lifestyle habits, and body type. Symptoms such as hot flashes, night sweats and weight gain can be very frustrating, and can also be signals of the need for lifestyle changes necessary for healthy aging.

After menopause, it can become too late to turn back the clock on chronic diseases such as artery thickening and obesity. I challenge you to take advantage of being a woman who is in the know and use the W*A*I*Pointes™ program to ensure you have a smooth transition and an awesome future.

In this chapter, I offer you a wide variety of tools to help you on your journey to health and wellness, including simple shifts in your daily routine and tips for creating yummy and healthy meals for you and your family. I hope they inspire you to create a lifetime of healthy makeovers. These short, but significant tips are designed to help you jump start your health and wellness makeover—NOW!

Are you getting what you need from your health care provider?

When is the last time your doctor asked you how you were raised and what you thought of your aging parents as they went through midlife? Have you discussed your dreams for how you will live in your 50s and beyond? Have you talked about how hard it will be to live in your 60s and beyond? Have you talked about how it is hard to maintain an exercise schedule with your otherwise busy life, and how the back pain you have had since childbirth makes most exercises difficult? Did your doctor assess your risk of heart disease or cancer, and formulate a plan for dealing with such risks? Did your doctor ask how often you are intimate with your partner, and if it was working for the both of you? Did you talk about your new onset cyclical headaches and mood changes before your periods? And, did you discuss how the stress of a shaky financial future is keeping you up at night?

As a physician, I believe it is my job to look at you with a holistic view and see how everything about you has an impact on your health and ability to enjoy life.

Take a minute to think about your last annual physical exam. Perhaps you still see the doctor who delivered your children, or you have changed to a family practice physician or internal medicine doctor. You likely waited several months to get the appointment, and perhaps it was even rescheduled several times between the doctor's schedule and your own. Once you got to the office, you likely waited for some time both in the waiting room and then in the examination room. A good doctor will have reviewed your chart before coming in the door and will take the time to review with you any changes in your family history, in your life and in your health since your last visit. Following the update, your doctor should discuss recommended screenings and other preventative measures such as a mammogram, colonoscopy, and a panel of blood tests to measure your cholesterol, hormone and thyroid levels. As you two continue to talk, most physicians likely would feel there would be more to discuss, but time is running out. The physical exam would then happen, ending with a Pap smear, ovarian and rectal exam. Hopefully health goals are discussed before the visit is ended, and plans for follow-up on the tests ordered are discussed.

Hopefully, you, the patient, felt listened to, cared for, and confident that the basics had been covered. You were probably also thankful the Pap is over for another year. That is how I always feel after my exam. I leave the office knowing I am able to check a major "to do" off the list and also know my ovaries are not enlarged, my mammogram is ordered, and face the fact that I'm still ten pounds over my goal weight. I also know to expect to receive a postcard in the mail that my Pap and other tests were normal.

So, medical standards were met, basics were covered, contact with the health care system was made. Was my health improved? Am I more likely to live a long, productive and disease-free life? Did that 15-minute annual physical make me more likely to make good choices when I am hungry at 9:00 p.m., exercise when I'm tired, reduce my stress level, and so on? Current statistics—and personal accounts I hear from patients and women every day—would argue, no. Sure, the current standard of care for women in midlife addressed the basics. But there's no time allotted to dig deeper, to address a woman's physical, mental and spiritual health goals. After your doctor tells you that you need to lose 30 pounds, do you walk out with a plan in hand to transform your daily living habits and a promise to return the next year a new svelte and healthy you? Most likely not.

Ten Questions You Need to Ask Your Physician

If you're looking to get the most comprehensive treatment possible from your health care provider, here's a checklist of questions to get answered at your appointment:

1. What is my phase of ovarian function? (Am I still in reproductive phase, in perimenopause, or in menopause?)

2. What is your (the physician's) training in menopause? What is your training in gender specific medicine—as in how a woman is different than a man?

3. What is my risk for heart disease? For diabetes? For breast cancer? For bone weakness (osteoporosis)? For uterine cancer? For colon cancer? For depression? For not being good at coping? There are screening tools for all of these and more; knowledge is power.

4. What is my Body Mass Index? Is it healthy?

5. Will you measure my waist circumference? I know that over 35 inches is not healthy.

6. Can I have a copy of my lab test results? I need to know my numbers.

7. How much Vitamin D do I need? Calcium?

8. Should I be taking a baby aspirin?

9. If I have questions about my sex drive, who do you recommend I talk to? What about vaginal dryness, what treatments do you suggest?

10. Can I have a copy of my mammogram, including BI-RADS (Breast Imaging Reporting and Data System) score?

Beware of health practitioners who offer the quick answer, the instant fix, or the magic hormone pellet. They are smart enough to know that vulnerable, stressed, sleep-deprived women with no time to spend on themselves will easily spend whatever it takes to get better quickly. Using terms like "natural," these often self-trained experts offer unproven advice and treatment without evidence of safety or efficacy. To further their business, they make doctors with real credentials who offer evidence-based treatment options and discussions of risks and benefits sound like the villains.

A word of advice: Do your research, and start by looking at the money trail. If the practitioner profits from the sale of supplements and compounded medications, it should be seen as a red flag. Often your insurance will cover the services of health care providers who are credentialed in women's health, gynecology, and menopause. They work for a living, but do not make more money depending on how many medications they prescribe or tests they order.

Dr. Diana L. Bitner, MD, NCMP

The Top Ten Insights Gained From my Patients

Here are the top ten insights I've learned from watching my patients navigate a transformed midlife by practicing W*A*I*Pointes™ :

1. Every Sunday, before the week starts, get out your schedule, and with SEEDS™ in front of you, put your exercise SEEDS™ on the calendar: short workouts on the days with less time, one long workout a week on the day you have more time, and two medium workouts where you have at least a 30-minute window.

2. Schedule one five-minute stretching event a day.

3. For night sweats, plan a five-minute metered breathing session before bed.

4. Think about the time of the day when you overeat and be prepared -- for many, it is about 3:00 p.m. Have a snack, such as two cheese sticks and an apple, or 10 Wheat Thins ready to go. Instead of having coffee, first drink a glass of water and consider a cup of tea because it offers a similar feeling, but has less caffeine.

5. Practice three gratitudes with your family. One patient has her family members say what they are grateful for each night at dinner, and she reflects on this later during metered breathing.

6. Get connected with what you want. One patient's goal was to be HOT at 50, instead of being 20 lbs. overweight and tired like she was at 46. She did it by staying connected with that picture.

7. Start dressing in light pajamas, even if you are cold going to sleep. You will warm up under the covers, but not enough to trigger a hot flash or night sweat.

8. Be aware of your triggers. Get out your Symptomcircle (available on the website at truewomenshealth.com) and study it. One patient would carry it in her purse to remind her to avoid the hot flash triggers like too much coffee or over-scheduling herself, and was able to avoid the resultant anxiety.

9. One patient got in the habit of standing and guzzling her glasses of water. After three days, she felt more energy, and her kidneys got used to it and she did not have to empty her bladder all the time!

10. Put an apple and cheese stick in the car for the drive home from work or from picking the kids up from school. If you eat it before hitting the door, you are less likely to eat junk and more likely to feel available to help with homework or to get a healthy dinner going.

That Three Letter Word—Sex

When couples come to see me together the conversation usually turns to sex. If they do not bring it up, I do because it tends to be the issue that causes the most friction between many couples. Now, I am NOT a sex therapist, but I have learned that even asking the questions and allowing either partner to voice their concerns or complaints in front of the other can be very therapeutic.

Also of note, I often care for same-sex couples as well as heterosexual partners, and the same principles tend to apply—especially if hormone changes are occurring at different times for each of them.

The most common issue for women, from my clinical experience, tends to be a lack of desire to initiate sex, and men's most common complaint is that they are not having enough sex which leaves them feeling as though they have done something wrong or are no longer loved.

I then usually ask about the different aspects of sexual desire for each of them. The men usually agree they prefer to have sex at night when the house is quiet and the doors are locked, king of the castle stuff is done, all is safe and secure, and they feel that sex just seals the deal of a happy and secure household.

For women, nighttime tends to be the first time they have any downtime at all, and are just plain tired. Many women feel as if people have been asking things of them all day, and if they have young children, then they have been giving and being touched all day. Being touched at night when relaxing to sit and pay bills or watch a show can be the last thing they wish to happen. Other issues such as pain with intercourse, depression or anxiety, poor self image from weight gain, fear the kids will get up and interrupt sex, and unresolved conflict between a couple all add up to a mismatch in satisfaction with the frequency of sex or the quality of the interaction.

By sorting out the different aspects of libido, I try to make it more objective and see what small changes could be made to improve the situation. Men should be aware of the cycle timing, in that women might be more interested in the first 2-3 weeks after a period ends versus right before. They should be sensitive to the stress of the end of the day; be more willing to pitch in with household chores if they know by relieving stress, it might enamor them to their partner. Helping with the kids' bath or emptying the dishwasher can be the best foreplay!

For women, by addressing the issues of mood, self image, vaginal comfort, ability to have an orgasm, and partner conflict can be freeing to allow for discussion and resolution. Sometimes a female partner initiating sex in the morning when she is rested, prioritizing exercise, and asking for more help in the household can be a boost to her sex drive. Causes of pelvic pain can be addressed by ruling out vaginal infections such as yeast or bacterial vaginosis, skin conditions such as lichen sclerosis, and bladder conditions such as interstitial cystitis. Pelvic floor physical therapists are often instrumental in helping women resolve issues of chronic pelvic pain and pelvic muscle spasm, as well as incontinence and prolapse. Vaginal dryness can generally be resolved with local estrogen.

In summary, if sex is an issue, then ask for a discussion and get to the bottom of the problem.

Recharge Your Steps—and Stick With It

No time for exercise? Buy a pedometer and supercharge your daily steps, by keeping track of each and every one of them. Then amplify your routine by setting a goal.

My recommendation: Start with 5,000 steps a day with the goal of ramping that up to 10,000 steps per day. Nail your performance with a little help. You can walk in place; pick up a video and/or walk on a treadmill. Head outside: go for a walk, hop on a bicycle or count your steps walking around the office during a 10-minute lunch break.

When you are wearing the pedometer, it will be fun to see the steps add up! Every night, write it down in your W*A*I*Pointes™ journal. Keeping track of your steps with a pedometer will motivate you and give you a strong foundation for building up your health.

Account for It All

Keep track of nearly everything you do every day—from what you eat, to how much you walk, to how you feel. Record it in your W*A*I*Pointes™ journal and Life Action Plan.

Dr. Diana L. Bitner, MD, NCMP

Pen a New Fitness Plan

Create a fitness plan for each week that will sync with your schedule. One trick I learned: On Sunday nights, I look at my schedule for the week ahead and pen in a physical activity just as I would a meeting with the hospital administrators, or an appointment with a patient. By doing this, I prioritize my fitness just like I do everything else in my weekly schedule.

It works like this: On crazy days, I know I will not get to exercise. These are the days I am on a 24-hour shift at the hospital. I turn that into a pedometer day. On the days where I have 20 minutes or less to exercise, I do a short activity like lower body strength training and sit-ups, or 10 minutes on the bike in the basement and 5-10 minutes of stretching.

On days with more time, I put on the calendar something longer—either upper body free weights, which take about 25 minutes after a five-minute warm-up, or a 30-40 minute fast and furious bike workout with Lady Gaga on my iPad, while reading Oprah's latest issue. Once a week I make sure I have time for a long 60-minute workout. I feel like I really empty my liver of long-term sugar stores (glycogen), and it takes the rest of the week for my body to fill it back up, instead of my overflow of calories going to fat.

Everyone has their own fitness plan that works, but this may give you some ideas about how you can be creative—and weave exercise into your daily routine.

The cumulative effect matters. An example of a good weekly exercise plan (50 minutes per day):

- Monday – lower body and ab/core workout
- Tuesday – upper body workout
- Wednesday – interval training session

- Thursday – lower body and ab/core workout
- Friday – yoga/stretching
- Saturday – interval training session
- Sunday – long moderate aerobic workout

The point is that it I put it on my schedule, just like work, appointments or meetings. I am more likely to do it if it is there.

Stretch with Ease

One of the back-to-basics moves you need to make time for every day is to stretch. And, like everything else, you need to make stretching a priority by penning it into your schedule. In the morning before your shower, do two minutes, then before bed do five minutes. You should do these stretches every day, even if you do the same routine every night and every morning. Think long and lean!

Kickstart Your Eating Makeover by Planning Ahead

Do diet foods really help you lose weight? In my experience and that of my patients, I don't think so. I do think you need to do some menu planning to stave off the temptation to drive through the fast food lane and order a burger and fries.

One of the tricks I have found to eating healthy is to plan my menu for a week. It doesn't have to be fancy, but if you are planning it out, you are less likely to fail.

Here's a look at another typical weekly menu that's right for me and my family—and it may help inspire ideas for you to eat your way to stellar health, too:

- Breakfast: I have the same Ezekiel toast with non-sugar peanut butter and honey every morning in the car on the way to work, or a smoothie made of almond milk, frozen berries and bananas, and Brazil nuts.
- Mid-day snack: Repeat of breakfast.
- Lunch: A vegetable pocket, a whole wheat bread sandwich, or my favorite—a salad made of arugula, vegetarian chicken nuggets and hot brown rice with olive oil and salt.
- Mid-afternoon snack: An apple and peanut butter, or cheese sticks, or a banana with 10 nuts, water, and then coffee.
- Dinner: Whatever I make for the family, except on my plate I leave off the carbs. My favorite meal is a roasted vegetable salad. Then I add a dish with protein. It could be my famous turkey lasagna, but I take no more than a bite of the noodles and focus instead on the sauce and meat. Another idea: You can throw frozen peas into the microwave and heat up a veggie burger if your family is munching on a casserole or carb-heavy meal.

Create exceptions (mini treats for you): Friday night a treat from the local pizza place and half of a cold beer. Saturday, I go back to the weekday routine, with the exception of maybe a glass of wine with dinner with friends; and Sunday morning, I enjoy my family's favorite whole wheat blueberry banana pancakes with natural maple syrup, and a fried egg.

The idea I'm trying to share with you is that if you have a schedule of recipes in place, it makes it easier for you to stay true to healthy choices.

Lose Weight, Feel Great

Exercise is important to weight loss, but diet is critical. Burning 60 calories through exercise and then rewarding yourself with an extra

100 calories will tip the scale in the opposite direction. By reducing your caloric intake by 100 calories a day, you can lose an additional pound per month. Combined with the 0.5 lbs. per month you burned off with exercise, would result in a 1.5 pound weight loss in one month, or 18 pounds in one year. That is weight lost in a healthy manner that can be sustained for a lifetime, and won't be regained as soon as you "come off" the diet. By not restricting your calories too drastically, your body will be able to preserve its lean body mass.

Including exercise in your diet plan will increase your lean body mass. This is important because it is the lean body mass that is metabolically active, even while at rest. Increasing your lean body mass increases the number of calories you burn on a daily basis. This increases the amount of weight lost over time and makes it much easier to maintain your new weight once you hit your goal, because you are able to eat more calories to sustain your current weight. Get out there and get active. You'll be glad you did.

10 Simple Ways to Cut 100 Calories From Your Diet

1. Remove the skin from your poultry after cooking.

2. Use fruit spread instead of butter on your toast.

3. Use nonstick cooking spray instead of oil or butter for cooking.

4. Switch to low-fat dairy products including milk, yogurt and cheese.

5. Instead of salad dressing, try balsamic vinegar, rice vinegar, lemon juice, or use less dressing.

6. When making an omelette, only use one egg yolk.

7. Leave the cheese off your burger and add lettuce, tomato, onion and pickles instead.

8. Steam your vegetables instead of sautéing.

9. Skip the croutons.

10. Order two slices of cheese and veggie pizza.

Tips for Jump-starting a Personalized Blueprint of Achievable Ways to Manage and Mitigate Midlife

- Write down your picture of how you want to be. If it's different from how you are now, write down what changes you need to make.
- Commit to becoming the woman you aspire to be. If you are at the place you want to be now, and then commit to maintaining, even if life throws you curve balls.
- Tell your partner and/or a good friend your new awareness of your body's changes and what is hard for you.
- Fashion a diary or join the online W*A*I*Pointes™ where you can journal online and track your symptoms and your SEEDS™.
- Purge junk food from your house, work and car. Think of junk food as stopping you from becoming that healthy person you want to be.
- Examine your daily spaces for clutter; it can zap your energy, especially in the space where you get ready in the morning and in your closet space. Organize your underwear drawer, your socks, and your clothes. Simplify!

- Clean out your car, your desk where you pay bills, and your purse. Start fresh on the levels you can most easily control!
- Think how you can make the changes easy to remember, not easy to forget. Place reminder notes about your POS where you can see them. Put your vitamins where you will remember them -- calcium in the car, a water bottle ready to go, exercise clothes next to your bed. Little preparations can make all the difference!
- Have a midlife action plan buddy. Compare your POS and PIP; compare ways you will reach your POS together.
- Find a doctor or health care provider who can help support you on this journey. Go to the NAMS website (menopause.org) or Healthtap (healthtap.com) to find someone in your area who is knowledgeable about menopause and midlife wellness.
- Be grateful for a chance to move forward with healthy plans, knowing what to do! It is a once-in-a-lifetime chance to change your future for the better without gimmicks or big life changes. Put a journal next to your bed to write down what your three gratitudes are every day.

Tips for Beating Stress

- Participate in pleasurable activities.
- Talk with friends.
- Eat three nutritious meals a day.
- Focus on a diet that is low in fat, sodium, refined sugar, alcohol, and caffeine.
- Snack on healthy, crunchy foods, such as apples and raw carrots.
- Make time for regular, daily exercise.
- Find or renew a creative outlet or activity that fulfills mental and/or spiritual needs.

- Enjoy self-care activities such as a massage, pedicure, or even a leisurely bath.
- Try stress reduction and relaxation techniques, such as deep breathing and meditation.
- Get adequate sleep each night.
- Laugh as much as possible.
- Join a support group.
- Seek professional help, if necessary.

*From the North American Menopause Society

Chapter Eleven

A Man's Guide to Understanding Menopause

Think of this as a male-centric primer on what to expect when your wife/sister/mother is expecting, or experiencing, the stages of menopause.

Truths Women Want You To Know

- It's not your fault. Don't take it personally when the woman in your life is having a hard time coping. It is not about you and you didn't cause it.

- It's the real thing. Understand that the effects of hormones are powerful and real. Hormonal fluctuation can cause a sometimes baffling array of symptoms such as mood swings, depression, irritability, increased fatigue, diminished sex drive, physical discomfort during sex, less desire to initiate sex, sleep disruption, hot flashes and night sweats.

- If you can, take action. Use this time as an opportunity to work together to strengthen and heal your relationship, instead of allowing tension and troubles to continue to mount. Unfortunately, if there is stress in your relationship already, it can get worse.

- Be patient. Her moods may be difficult to read. You may not know if she wants a hug or is channeling her inner hermit, i.e. wants to be left alone. Sometimes she doesn't know what she wants. When things are calm, the two of you could come up with a fun signaling system. Create signs that spell it out, red for Time Out or blue for Hug, Please.

- Be a comfort. Bring her a cup of herbal tea, remind her to drink more water, draw a bath and keep the teenagers occupied. One of the tools I recommend (see Chapter Six) is Seven Essential Elements for Daily Success SEEDS™. Helping her incorporate these daily strategies into her life will make a big difference.

- Beat the temporary blues. Know that she does not like how she is feeling and is confused by it as well. Imagine if you played tennis and every week you did well, or you could play a pickup game whenever and wherever, and never had any physical complaints. Then, your knee starts to ache more and more each time, until one time it is bad enough you have to cancel a game. You go to the doctor, and he tells you that you have arthritis and will have to limit how many games you play. That's how she feels when she's served up the news about her body changing.

- It IS a big deal. Often men want to believe it isn't happening, and for that matter, she wishes it would go away, too. You may want to read up on menopause to learn more about what is happening to her physically, mentally and emotionally. Understand that she feels her body is betraying her. Her high energy level seems to be tanking. She may feel fatigued; less inspired and have less incentive to get things done. She may feel more irritable toward you and less patient with herself. She's wondering why her body suddenly feels as if it's on fire (and not in a good way).

- For a moment, imagine what a hot flash feels like—you're in the desert at high noon dressed in a ski suit, wrapped in an Arctic weather-worthy down coat and covered with a blanket. Now imagine that heat coming over you in a flash, as you're in the middle of a staff meeting, on the train home or standing in the checkout line at the supermarket. Your cheeks are turning hot pink, and sweat is pouring out of you. Not so pretty, right? And that's just one of the symptoms.

- It's OK to feel frustrated. She is as sleep deprived as you both were after your first child was born (although she may have been more sleep deprived then, too). She felt groggy all day, had to put on her game face at work (see hot flash above), stopped at the grocery store on the way home, made dinner, arranged the kids' schedules, set up the teacher conference and finally got into bed. And then you're feeling frisky and ready for sex.

- You don't have to fix it. Many men respond to their wives as if they are sick, need to get treated, and then it will be over. There's no magic pill. Don't treat her like a broken object you have to fix. Just be supportive and understanding.

- When to seek help. Major depression, erratic or manic behavior cannot be explained away by changing hormone levels. If her mood swings become seismic shifts or if you see physical symptoms such as dizziness, frequent faintness or notice symptoms that signal something serious, call her doctor.

Final Thoughts from Diana

At 48, I am just starting to understand my path, and see how everything in my life has added up to who I am and what I have to offer. All the people in my life and my experiences have played a part.

When I get caught up in worry, or drama, or allow doubt to overshadow intuition, my heart and forebrain close down, and I say and do things I shouldn't. How do I keep an open heart and thus stay connected to my purpose and my true self? I, for the time being, will close my eyes for a second to smell an open fire and see a cozy scene of good friends, and remember a feeling of calm. After being in that place for a minute or two, I take the situation at hand and do my best to stay true.

I am a woman who is blessed with a life that fits me well. But it did not just happen. My life has been marked by bright moments of love, success and clarity, and also by times of fear, abandonment and uncertainty. I have dreamed of being a doctor since a young age, and I am thankful for inborn focus which has kept me on track. Learning to own my power has been crucial and requires continued daily practice.

I wrote this book because I have expertise and insight to share, and I am still sometimes surprised that my approach to patient care works time and time again. For over 20 years, I have been blessed to be included in women's lives at their most important moments. Each woman and her situation is unique, from pregnancies and births, health histories and conditions such as diabetes and cancer, and crises of postpartum depression, to cheating husbands and emergencies like unwanted hysterectomies in women who couldn't have children. I have had to learn to wear many hats, switching between surgeon, psychologist, mother, and friend.

Using the W*A*I* Pointes™ principles has made it easier to see how every aspect of a woman's life fits together to make her well or unwell as she ages. A big part of my practice is seeing women for their annual exam. More and more, I have seen how these appointments turn into W*A*I* Pointes™ visits.

Wherever you are in your mid-life journey—at the starting line, still walking or running, or already across the menopause finish line, you know your body and your life are changing. Very few of us want, or wish, to age or grow old.

What's the alternative? Short of finding a genie in a bottle, a working time travel machine or that elusive fountain of youth, you can't stop aging, but you can choose how you'll go about it. Choose to age gracefully, age smartly, age with energy, vitality, drive, ambition and happiness, age with a sense of adventure. Use the change of life to change your life. Use it as a ticket to the best time of your life, a catalyst for personal transformation, an opportunity to reenergize your body, mind and soul. And there is no time like the present.

As a physician, I have a unique opportunity to share the journey with my patients, to support them and cheer them on. As a healer, I feel fulfilled when I see a patient jettison bad habits, clear the clutter from her life and embrace daily lifestyle changes that will keep her healthier and happier in the years to come. As a 48-year-old wife, mom and a woman who, just like you, is struggling with my own hot flashes and midlife health challenges, I am also a fellow traveler on this midlife journey.

I wrote this book because I couldn't find a book or resource that fully and completely incorporated traditional medicine with a full body, mind and spirit holistic approach that talks about nutrition and phase of ovarian function, that asks women to revisit their goals and to imagine the future they want, to create a picture of self that will turn into a self-fulfilling "prophecy." Frustration was the mother of this invention.

As I've stated throughout, my vision and goal in writing this book is to help you age healthfully and vibrantly without chronic illness, cancer, or pain by using your dreams and goals as motivation to make good daily choices.

And now that you've figured out your Place in Process (PIP), developed your Picture of Self (POS), created your Life Action Plan and completed the questionnaires, I invite you to venture onto the website (truewomenshealth.com), to delve deeper and discover more tools to help you refine your path to wellness. I invite you to meet new friends as we build a community of women on the verge of changing midlife.

Enjoy the journey,

Dr. Diana L. Bitner, MD, NCMP

Acknowledgements

As I re-read this book before final sign off, I am struck by the thought of all life's lessons which have brought me to this place. I am indebted to my many teachers throughout the years, starting with grade school. As all of us do, I have had many moments of epiphany which opened my world and took me to the next level. Many situations were difficult, but served as gifts in the long run.

I am grateful to my family and friends who have supported my truth in needing to write this book, and understanding the need for time and effort which were involved in this work, which does not feel like work.

I am forever indebted to the girls and women who have been my patients—for the trust given me by them, their families and referring physicians—to care for them during pregnancies, delivery of their children, surgeries, treatment of gynecological concerns, and during the many changes and symptoms of midlife and menopause. I love my day job and have been given more than I gave.

I am grateful to my partners at work—eight very busy physicians with families and lives who took extra calls so I could complete the W*A*I*Pointes™ Pilot study and change my practice focus to midlife and menopause medicine. I could not have done this without your support.

The leadership at MMPC, starting with John Mackeigen, Dom Federico, Allyn Lebster, Deidra McClellend, Ted Inman, Mike Puff, Phil Hoekstra, Greg Gadbois—the list goes on—who, before we merged with Spectrum Health, supported my passion for women's health and the W*A*I*Pointes™ Pilot study with timely lessons and financial and moral support. Since the merge, I thank my physician bosses Rick Leach and Julian "Skip" Schinck for their support, and the Spectrum Health Innovations team, namely Brett Mulder, Mike Miller, and former Director Kris White, as well as the Spectrum Health Research and Marketing teams. Michael Gouin-Hart, you are a fantastic medical writer, and I am indebted to Cynthia Giles who took painstaking care with data collection and analysis for the W*A*I*Pointes™ Pilot study. I thank Beth Reed for her excellent care of patients and attention to detail during the W*A*I*Pointes™ Pilot study.

I thank the NAMS leadership including Margery Gass, JoAnn Manson, JoAnn Pinkerton, Jan Shifren, Pauline Maki, Jim Simon, Nanette Santoro, Michelle Warren, and especially Bob Wild—my mentor in the NAMS menopause research mentor-mentee program—for their dedication to gender-specific medicine, seeing the potential in my ideas, and teaching me the importance of good research principles and statistics.

To my assistant, Jill Cross, who keeps me grounded, moving in the right direction and helping to make sure it all happens.

To the newly formalized executive team of truewomenshealth.com, thank you for your die-hard support of the principles of W*A*I*Pointes™ and believing in the concept since day one. We are going to make a difference!

George Sopko, thank you for your example and stories of perseverance, for seeing the potential in my vision for women's health, and reminding me "this IS the NIH."

To the editor of this book, the blog, and numerous articles, Barb Rickard, thank you for your incredible attention to detail and gifted word-smithing. Yes, I am the author, you are the writer. I am ok with this.

To Tricia, the publisher extraordinaire and owner of Splattered Ink Press, thank you for your vision to create such a personable business model to allow authors like me to be heard, and for your encouragement and professionalism. I look forward to working together frequently in the future.

Works Cited

Chapter Three

There is much work and research ongoing around the concept of coping. I have gained insight from articles about the COPE Score, reference: Carver, CS, Scheier, MF, and Weintraub JK 1989, Assessing Coping Strategies: A theoretically based approach; Journal of Personality and Social Psychology; 56, 267-283

PHQ-9 is a nine question test used to assess for symptoms of depression. The reference is Kroenke K, Spitzer R, Williams W. The PHQ-9: Validity of a brief depression severity measure. JGIM, 2001, 16:606-616

The first book I read by Suze Orman was <u>9 Steps to Financial Freedom, Practical and Spiritual Steps So You Can Stop Worrying</u>, Three Rivers Press, 2006. It made a strong impression on me and helped me face my fear of money.

Chapters Four and Five

This chapter includes evidence-based and validated risk scores which I did NOT develop. They are publicly available for use.

The presidential fitness score for adult women is available at <u>adultfitnesstest.org</u> (accessed July 11, 2014).

Description of how to correctly obtain waist circumference measurements is at <u>cdc.gov/healthyweight/assessing/Index.html</u> and a chart of what risks are best known to be associated with elevated waist circumference can be found on the NIH site nhlbi.nih.gov/health/public/heart/obesity/lose_wt/bmi_dis.htm.

For cancer risk assessment, there are widely available stratification scores. None perfectly predict risk for the population or individual, but at least get us thinking and acting on modifiable risk factors. For breast cancer I use the Gail Model. It can be found at cancer.gov/bcrisktool/.

For colon and lung cancer, I use the Washington University Risk tools at www.yourdiseaserisk.wustl.edu/YDRDefault.aspx?ScreenControl=YDRGeneral&ScreenName=YDRCancer_Index.

Heart disease is the number one killer of women and many of the causative factors are preventable!! A female- or gender-specific risk stratification tool is the Reynolds Score, and can be found at reynoldsriskscore.org.

When I was thinking about how to structure the risk score for Income Security, my personal banker and friend Nancy Monterusso was very helpful and I am indebted to her for her help and guidance.

Chapter Five

The stages of transition through stages of aging can be very confusing when hormones are involved. A workshop was convened and sponsored by the North American Menopause Society by thought leaders to make terminology consistent to allow for research and clinical conversation around this topic.

While I call the area of wellness "Phases of Ovarian Function," it is a scoring system based on the nomenclature developed by the workshop, first in 2001 and then re-confirmed in 2011. The flowchart is a clinical tool I developed to make the staging chart more user-friendly by my patients, and has not been endorsed by the authors or NAMS. The reference paper is *Executive summary of the Stages of Reproductive Aging Workshop D 10: Addressing the unfinished agenda of staging reproductive aging,* Sioban D. Harlow, Ph.D.,a Margery Gass, M.D., N.C.M.P.,b Janet E. Hall, M.D.,c Roger Lobo, M.D.,d Pauline Maki, Ph.D.,e Robert W. Rebar, M.D.,f Sherry Sherman, Ph.D.,g Patrick M. Sluss, Ph.D., and Tobie J. de Villiers, M.B.Ch.B., F.R.C.O.G., F.C.O.G.(SA),i for the STRAW þ 10 Collaborative Group, Fertility and Sterility® Vol. 97, No. 4, April 2012 0015-0282 Copyright ©2012 American Society for Reproductive Medicine

For more information on menopause, to find a menopause practitioner in your area, and to learn about the North American Menopause Society (NAMS), go to menopause.org.

DEXA is an acronym to describe the tool and process of measuring bone density and attempting to predict a woman's risk of fracture. The FRAX score goes steps further to use additional risk factors for a woman in menopause in addition to the DEXA to predict fracture risk and gauge whether pharmaceutical therapy could be indicated. The FRAX score is publicly available at www.atshef.ac.uk/FRAX/tool.aspx?country=9.

The Reynolds Score has been developed and compared to the Framingham Score and does a better job in classifying women's heart disease risk. The score itself for individual use is available at reynoldsriskscore.org and a comprehensive article about its development and use is found in the journal Circulation:

Cook NR, Paynter NP, Eaton CB, Manson JE, Martin LW, Robinson JG, Rossouw JE, Wassertheil-Smoller S, Ridker PM. *Comparison of the Framingham and Reynolds risk scores for global cardiovascular risk prediction in the multiethnic Women's Health Initiative.* Circulation. 2012;125:1748-1756.

Chapter Six

The topic of water consumption is controversial. I have heard all different recommendations stated by experts with total conviction at national conventions. Each woman will find her balance. Being aware of the side effects of too much or more commonly, too little, is the first step to taking control of your health and symptoms. There is sparse data to determine an exact amount necessary to optimize wellness. It is accepted that cold water can temper a hot flash if it occurs; for more information see a benchmark article: Freedman RR. Pathophysiology and treatment of menopausal hot flashes. Semin Reprod Med. May 2005; 23(2):117-125.

Sleep requirements can also be different for each individual, but it is accepted that most require 7-8 hours per night for optimal function, but many aged 40-55 report sleeping less than 7 hours per night. uptodate.com, accessed July 11, 2014.

Sleep requirements and sleep disturbance through the menopause transition is a hot area of research, and sleep deprivation is thought to affect symptoms such as mood and hot flashes, and also risk for chronic disease.

Metered breathing and paced respirations have been studied in the treatment of hot flashes and night sweats by many different groups, each with different methods. The method and timing discussed here were piloted in the W*A*I*Pointes™ Pilot study, "A clinical intervention to reduce central obesity and menopausal symptoms in women aged 35-55," Bitner DB and Wild RA, in press, Menopause.

The quotes from Baron Baptiste are from his video *Journey into Power Baptiste Power Yoga*, Level II available at baronbaptiste.com, accessed July 11, 2014.

Vitamin D is a complex subject and dosing recommendations are under review in a benchmark study by Dr. JoAnn Manson; information is available at vitalstudy.com; information here quoted in part from the textbook <u>Menopause Practice: A Clinician's Guide</u>, 4th Edition, 2010 published by NAMS.

More information on glycemic index of food is available in the book <u>Sugarbusters! Cut Sugar to Trim Fat</u> by Leighton, Bethea, Andrews, and Balant, Ballantine, 1998.

More information is available on dietary fiber requirements at mayoclinic.com, accessed July 11, 2014.

The science behind relaxation practice has been well described in the book <u>Relaxation Response</u> by Herbert Benson MD, William Morrow 1975.

<u>Chapter Eight</u>

Hormone replacement is a complicated topic and many statements of recommendation guidelines are available at menopause.org. The WHI study was unfortunately hyped by the media and the data was misused, and essentially deprived many women from hormone replacement therapy unnecessarily. The WHI helped to inform us who can have hormones and when, for whom hormones are not safe, and how long it is safe to stay on hormone replacement therapy. We are now interested in comparing different regimens, oral versus patch, and this is being looked at in the ongoing research study called the Kronos Early Estrogen Replacement Trial; information is available at keepstudy.org.

I also keep an active blog which can be found at spectrumhealthblogs.org/menopause and will update the blog regarding HRT as new information becomes available.

There are many resources available for non-hormonal therapies and CAM Therapeutics, but the resource I most frequently turn to is the

Dr. Diana L. Bitner, MD, NCMP

<u>Menopause Practice, A Clinician's Guide</u> 2010 4th Edition, published by NAMS because of the evidence-based approach and references.

Recommended Reading and Resources

Compiled from the recommendations of my patients – and my own favorites, this collection of books will also help you celebrate your mid-life journey, and inspire and guide you along the way.

Williamson, Marianne. The Age of Miracles: Embracing the New Midlife
Northrup, Christiane M.D. The Wisdom of Menopause: Creating Physical and Emotional Health and Healing During the Change
Jonekos, Staness with Wendy Klein MD. The Menopause Makeover: The Ultimate Guide to Taking Control of Your Health and Beauty During Menopause

Overall Health & Wellness

Peeke, Pamela, M.D., M.P.H., F.A.A.C.P. Body for Life for Women: A Woman's Plan for Physical and Mental Transformation
Roizen, Michael F. M.D. Real Age: Are You as Young as You Can Be?
Ramsland, Marcia. Simplify Your Life
Christiane Northrup M.D. Women's Bodies, Women's Wisdom: Creating Physical and Emotional Health and Healing
Michael F. Roizen, Michael F. M.D. and Mehmet C. Oz, M.D. You: Staying Young: The Owner's Manual for Extending Your Warranty

Physical Fitness

Cruise, Jorge. <u>8 Minutes in the Morning: A Simple Way to Shed Up to 2 Pounds a Week Guaranteed</u>
Baptiste, Baron. <u>Journey Into Power: How to Sculpt Your Ideal Body, Free Your True Self, and Transform Your Life with Yoga</u> (and other books)

Nutrition

Calorie King. <u>Calorie, Fat, and Carbohydrate Counter</u>
Berley, Peter. <u>Fresh Food Fast: Delicious, Seasonal Vegetarian Meals in Under an Hour</u>
<u>The New Mayo Clinic Cookbook. Eating Well for Better Health</u>
Steward, H. Leighton, Morrison C. Bethea, M.D., Sam S. Andrews, M.D., & Luis A. Balart, M.D. <u>Sugar Busters! Cut Sugar to Trim Fat</u>
Roizen, Michael F. M.D. and Mehmet C. Oz, M.D. <u>You on a Diet: The Owner's Manual for Waist Management</u>

Emotional Health

Lesser, Elizabeth. <u>Broken Open: How Difficult Times Can Help Us Grow</u>
Bradberry, Travis and Jean Greaves. <u>The Emotional Intelligence Quick Book: Everything you need to know to put your EQ to Work</u>
Goleman, Daniel. <u>Emotional Intelligence: Why It Can Matter More Than IQ</u>
Borysenko, Joan Ph.D. <u>It's Not the End of the World: Developing Resilience in Times of Change</u>

Financial Security

Bach, David. <u>Smart Women Finish Rich: 9 Steps to Achieving Financial Security and Funding Your Dreams</u>

Web Link Resources for Your Mid-life Journey

North American Menopause Society--www.menopause.org
Women's Health Information from the Federal Government--www.womenshealth.gov
Breast Cancer Risk Assessment Tool--www.cancer.gov/bcrisktool
Dr. Diana L. Bitner, MD at Spectrum Health Medical Group - www.shmg.org/womenshealthnetwork
Assessing your risk of heart disease and stroke--www.reynoldsriskscore.org
Financial advice--www.jeanchatzky.com
Sex and Intimacy www.lauraberman.com

More Resources

If you are looking for a menopause physician in your area, check out The North American Menopause Society (menopause.org). There is a search feature on this website for those women in the United States or Canada who are searching for physicians and other health care providers interested in helping them manage their health through menopause and beyond. Those who have passed a competency examination leading to the prestigious credential of NAMS Menopause Practitioner are noted in the displayed results.

About the Author

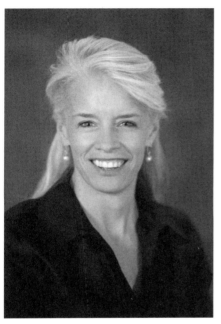

Dr. Diana L. Bitner, MD, NCMP, Director of The Spectrum Health Medical Group Women's Health Network and Certified Menopause Practitioner for the North American Menopause Society.

Women's Midlife health expert Dr. Diana L. Bitner, MD, NCMP, provides transformative tips for women to choose the healthiest road into the middle years and beyond in her new book, *I Want to Age Like That! Healthy Aging through Midlife and Menopause.*

Through her private practice, the book and as Director of The Spectrum Health Medical Group Women's Health Network, Diana teaches women how to age with vigor and grace. A Certified Menopause Practitioner for the North American Menopause Society, Diana empowers women to make lifestyle changes, educates them about the physical changes of midlife, and arms them with tools adapt their lifestyles and healthy, balanced lives into the future. She also provides methods and tips to tackle nutritional deficiencies, weight gain and low energy, plus a formula for reinventing, and creating a roadmap for living healthy with new dreams and renewed passion.

Drawing upon her 20-plus years as an OB/GYN and Certified Menopause Practitioner, delivering hundreds of babies, diagnosing and treating all manners of gynecological problems, challenges and illnesses, she's learned that many women today feel uniformed, disempowered and unable to make daily health choices in support of their personal goals and aspirations. Now, she offers new and insightful information for women in midlife – and the health care community about daily health choices that can have long-lasting effects on health.

In addition to being a physician and health advocate, Diana, 48, of Grand Haven, MI, is a wife, mother of three, avid cook and dog-lover. She graduated from medical school at Wayne State University in 1992 and with a B.S. in Biology and Chemistry in 1988 from Central Michigan University.

Dr. Bitner was a regular contributor on the SiriusXM Radio 107 show, Broadminded Broads from 8 a.m. to 10 a.m. EST and a frequent guest on Michigan local TV.

To see a short video of Diana discussing healthy aging, visit: http://www.woodtv.com/dpp/eightwest/Healthy_Aging.

"I wrote this book to help women prepare themselves physically and mentally for the road in and out of Menopause and Midlife. As a physician who's spent her life dealing with women's issues, I've always been passionate about translating what I know into language my patients can understand. I advocate do-it-yourself preventive medicine. By that I mean adapting your habits and lifestyle so you can travel along the path of wellness well into the future."

The book puts all this together and is about you remembering and reconnecting with that future self you wish to be, and using the best of medical wisdom to become her, despite life's challenges. I am grateful I have experience and knowledge to share and am humbled and grateful to think it might help even one woman avoid a heart attack or breast cancer or to have additional high quality years of activity and joy. Thank you for the opportunity to be a part of your life!"